Child Labour: A Public Health Perspective

Edited by

Anaclaudia G. Fassa

David L. Parker

Thomas J. Scanlon

OXFORD
UNIVERSITY PRESS

OXFORD
UNIVERSITY PRESS

Great Clarendon Street, Oxford OX2 6DP
Oxford University Press is a department of the University of Oxford.
It furthers the University's objective of excellence in research, scholarship,
and education by publishing worldwide in

Oxford New York

Auckland Cape Town Dar es Salaam Hong Kong Karachi
Kuala Lumpur Madrid Melbourne Mexico City Nairobi
New Delhi Shanghai Taipei Toronto

With offices in

Argentina Austria Brazil Chile Czech Republic France Greece
Guatemala Hungary Italy Japan Poland Portugal Singapore
South Korea Switzerland Thailand Turkey Ukraine Vietnam

Oxford is a registered trade mark of Oxford University Press
in the UK and in certain other countries

Published in the United States
by Oxford University Press Inc., New York

First published 2010

British Library Cataloguing in Publication Data
Data available

Library of Congress Cataloging in Publication Data
Data available

Typeset in Minion by Glyph International, Bangalore
Printed in Great Britain
on acid-free paper by
the MPG Books Group, Bodmin and King's Lynn

ISBN 978–0–19–955858–2

10 9 8 7 6 5 4 3 2 1

Oxford University Press makes no representation, express or implied, that the drug dosages in this book are correct. Readers must therefore always check the product information and clinical procedures with the most up-to-date published product information and data sheets provided by the manufacturers and the most recent codes of conduct and safety regulations. The authors and the publishers do not accept responsibility or legal liability for any errors in the text or for the misuse or misapplication of material in this work. Except where otherwise stated, drug dosages and recommendations are for the non-pregnant adult who is not breastfeeding.

To Ana, Pedro and Gabriel
To Mary
To Chesca, Louisa, Kathleen, Aidan and Sean
And to child labourers all over the world who are a reminder of the need to build a more just world.

Foreword

Children have always worked. Until the industrial revolution of the late 18th century most of this work was focused around the home – caring for younger children, tending crops and animals, gathering or preparing food, building protective shelters, or other work necessary for continued daily existence. The evolution of guilds in the middle of the last millennium associated with the apprenticing of children to tradesmen was probably the first major movement away from family-based work. Although guilds provided work for children outside of the family setting, the setting and work of an apprentice was not always in the best interest of the child. Yet social prohibitions concerning child labour were few.

With the dawn of the industrial revolution, dramatic changes in agriculture, manufacturing, and mining were associated with equally dramatic changes to every aspect of daily life. For children this meant increasing engagement in work away from family, work that was often dangerous, arduous, and long. This work occurred in industrial operations such as the textile industry, in mining, and even in the military and child prostitution.

Social attention concerned with misuse of children gradually grew with Victorian era concern both for child welfare and education. In the 21st century attention has certainly been focused on the most heinous and tragic ways in which children are forced into completely unacceptable work in the military or in the sex trades. And increasingly we have identified and condemned employment in the most hazardous work where children are at high risk of serious or fatal injury. We have also begun to address, as inappropriate, work that exposes children to toxic agents causing both acute and chronic poisoning. Industrialized nations and some developing nations have codified protections in labour or public health law. Enforcement of these laws, however, has been quite variable. And while children have gained some protections from the worst working conditions in developed nations even there, problems persist.

Beyond protecting children from hazardous or forced labour, concern has been raised with the amount of work – how working long or inappropriate hours interferes with the critical education of our children. As well, there is great concern with efforts to justify child labour as economically essential to the family. This despite the studies that show families that suffer the worst poverty are most likely to expect their children to work to assist in family survival. Rather than a route out of poverty, these are the families that are being trapped in a never-ending spiral to the bottom of the economic pyramid.

Finally there are those in the industrialized world who make a case for work by older children as part of the maturation process where lessons for a successful adulthood are learned. In the United States, it has been suggested that children between 14 and 17 should be given work opportunities to learn about responsibility, punctuality, engaging with people, and money management. While these may be useful and practical skills the work offered to youth generally is not designed to promote development of these skills. In fact, there is little evidence that gaining such skills at an early age is necessary to success.

As societies have come to focus quite serious attention on child labour, the many and varied issues related to control or elimination of child labour have proved difficult to solve. National, regional, and local attention is still needed to promote appropriate work, which is accepted voluntarily, and without adverse effect on education or development. Actually, it is highly desirable to find a new framework to understand child labour, both the problem and successful routes to its solution.

A number of scholarly works have been concerned with the problems of modern-day child labour and how best to promote child growth, development, and education in the face of the drivers that lead or force children to work. What is unusual about the treatment of the subject presented here is that we are provided with a framework that goes well beyond viewing the issue as a problem just about children, regardless of how substantive and well researched that view might be.

Rather the authors choose to approach child labour as a human concern that both affects and is affected by the entire community, and not just the individual child or the family. By using a human rights-based public health model we are provided with a fundamental life course perspective on a central concern of modern society. A comprehensive understanding of the role of children within the structural, social, and cultural context of society permits us to see the relationships between the role of work for children and the future health of the societies in which they are born.

The treatment of the subject is neither simplistic nor simple. We are reminded that there is no single way to view the role of children and work in every society. Instead we are challenged to recognize the fundamental differences in cultural and historical views of the place of children in a society. This is necessary if we are to promote appropriate and honest engagement of communities to examine and alter, as necessary, the place of early work in the lives of children.

The task is not easy and the evidence for success is not great. But this monograph is greatly enriched by case studies that show how substantially different approaches are being tested at the local, regional, and national level. The ultimate lesson is that there is no single correct approach for a society in addressing the complexities of child labour.

David H. Wegman
Professor Emeritus
Department of Work Environment
University of Massachusetts Lowell

Contents

Contributors

Anita Amorim
Senior Policy Advisor on United Nations Reform, External Relations and Partnerships Branch, International Labour Organization Geneva, Switzerland

Raheela Ayub
Occupational Medicine Resident, HealthPartners Clinic, Minneapolis, USA

Jo Boyden
Reader in Development Studies, Department of International Development, University of Oxford, UK

Charita L. Castro
Division Chief for Operations and Research, Office of Child Labor, Forced Labor and Human Trafficking, United States Department of Labor, Washington, DC, USA

Renata M. Coimbra Libório
São Paulo State University (UNESP) Presidente Prudente, São Paulo, Brazil

Eric V. Edmonds
Associate Professor of Economics, Dartmouth College, IZA and NBER Hanover, New Hampshire, USA

Anaclaudia G. Fassa
Associate Professor, Federal University of Pelotas, Brazil

Susan Gunn
Senior Technical Advisor, Hazardous Child Labour, International Labour Organization, Geneva, Switzerland

Lisa Ide
Medical Director, Employee Occupational Health, Fairview Health Services, Minneapolis, USA

Ana Lúcia Kassouf
Professor, University of São Paulo, Piracicaba, Brazil

Natalie W. Kohner
Attorney, Anderson, Helgen, Davis and Nissen, Minneapolis, USA

Silvia H. Koller
Centre for Pscyhological Studies of Street Children, Federal University of Rio Grande do Sul, Porto Alegre, Brazil

Barbara C. Lee
Marshfield Clinic Research Foundation, Marshfield, Wisconsin, USA

Mary E. Miller
Child Labor – Teen Worker Supervisor, Department of Labor and Industries, Tacoma, Washington State, USA

Virginia Morrow
Reader in Childhood Studies,
Institute of Education,
University of London,
London, UK

Philista Onyango
African Network for the Prevention and Protection against Child Abuse and Neglect (ANPPCAN)
Head office, Kenya, Africa

Ana Maria Osorio
Assistant Regional Director – Latin America,
US Food and Drug Administration,
US Department of Health and Human Services, Santiago, Chile

Nadine Osseiran
Programme Officer,
International Programme on the Elimination of Child Labour,
International Labour Organization
Geneva, Switzerland

David L. Parker
Epidemiologist and Physician, HealthPartners and Park Nicollet Clinic,
Minneapolis, Minnesota, USA

Noemi Miyasaka Porro
Adjunct Professor, Federal University of Pará,
Belém, Brazil

David Post
Professor of Education,
Pennsylvania State University,
Pennsylvania, USA

Thomas J. Scanlon
Consultant in Public Health,
Honorary Research Fellow,
Institute of Child Health,
London, UK

Nina Smith
Executive Director,
RugMark Foundation,
Washington, DC, USA

Amaryllis T. Torres
Dean,
College of Social Work and Community Development,
University of Philippines,
Diliman, Quezon City, Philippines

David Weissbrodt
Regents Professor,
University of Minnesota Law School,
Minneapolis, Minnesota, USA

Chapter 1

Introduction

Anaclaudia G. Fassa, David L. Parker, and Thomas J. Scanlon

Child labour has been a concern within the international community for almost a century and significantly longer at country level. The earliest regulation of child labour dates to 1284 when a statute adopted by a guild of Venetian glass makers forbade the employment of children in certain dangerous activities within the glass trade. However, although child labour is not unique to the current era, in more recent times as data have improved, the extent of the problem has become more apparent.

In 2004, the International Labour Organization (ILO) estimated that there were 211 million working children aged 5–14 years[1] around the world [1]. While this represents a reduction from 250 million working children in 2000, neither estimate includes children who have been trafficked or are in armed conflict, forced or bonded labour; prostitution or pornography; or other illicit work activities, such as drug trafficking. In addition, in many countries, especially in sub-Saharan Africa, war, natural disasters, and HIV and AIDS, have left children homeless, or as heads of households, responsible for younger siblings.

The last two decades have seen a discernible switch in policies with regard to child labour. These have gone from being centred on the adoption of a universal minimum age for child work, to the identification and elimination of harmful child work. This has been demonstrated by the reduced focus on ILO

[1] Three groups of working children are identified in ILO figures: (1) Economically active children/working children refers to children aged 5–17 years who undertake a least 1 hour of economic work per week; (2) Child labour refers to children aged 5–14 years engaged in at least 1 hour of economic work per week; (3) Children in hazardous work refers to children aged 5–17 years engaged in at least 1 hour of economic activity per week in occupations deemed hazardous, including children working in mining and construction, working with heavy machinery, exposed to pesticides, or working 43 hours or more a week.

(Minimum Age) Convention 138 and the almost universal acceptance of ILO (Elimination of the Worst Forms of Child Labour) Convention 182.

Using a rights-oriented public health model of child labour, this book seeks to synthesize a discussion on the key causes and consequences of child labour in the early 21st century. These are discussed in terms of the individual child, as well as the wider context of the family and community. A rights-oriented public health model adds several dimensions to the discussion of child labour. It makes exploitative and abusive work not only a labour market or health problem, but also an issue of human dignity. It insists that remedies preserve the rights of every child to be provided for, to be protected, and to participate in decisions related to his or her wellbeing. It accounts for the relationship between individuals and their community. It makes the connection between health, economics, education, social values, and legislation. Finally, it helps communities, and programme and policy makers identify comprehensive solutions to the burdens that child labour places on children, families, and the community.

Contributing authors have been asked to frame their contributions in the context of this model of child labour. Case studies have been selected and are presented on the basis of their relationship to the health of individual children and their communities. It is not the case, however, that there is consensus among contributing authors on the causes of, consequences of, and solutions to child labour. Nor this book is free from paradox. For example, the economics chapter explores the idea of compensated hazardous child work, the rights chapter includes a discussion on the right to work, and the case study of coco babaçu workers in northern Brazil illustrates how hazardous child labour can define the identity of a community, and how attempts to eradicate it can be interpreted as an infringement of the rights of traditional communities.

The presence of such paradoxes and the global acceptance that eradication of all child labour is unlikely should not be interpreted as a meek acceptance that short of ending the unconditional worst forms, the world should simply accept child labour. Similarly, the lack of direct evidence for the harm that child labour inflicts on children, families, and communities – due largely to a host of difficulties in undertaking good research, should not be misunderstood as evidence that most child labour does little harm. What emerges from this book is the opposite.

We, as editors, are grateful to the authors for their time and expertise in contributing to this book. Having set out our rights-oriented public health model of child labour, we may have asked them to review their contributions more often than was anticipated. They have, however, done so most graciously.

The result, we hope, is a coherent text that offers the reader an overview of child labour and a model of child labour which will assist in defining and identifying harmful child work, and can contribute to framing the policy response by which all working children will be better served.

Reference

1 Hagemann F, Diallo Y, Etienne A, Mehran F (2006). *Global child labour trends: 2000 to 2004*. Geneva: ILO.

Part 1

Child labour profile

Chapter 2

An overview of child labour statistics

Charita L. Castro

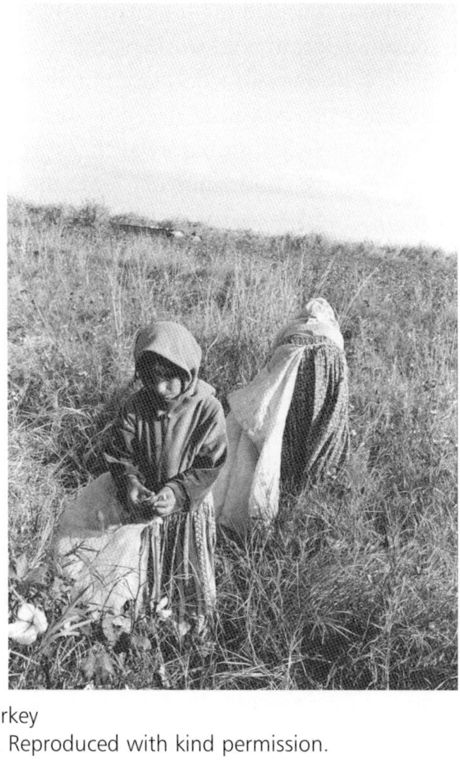

Picking cotton, Turkey

Introduction

In the field of international human rights, the measurement of social phenomena with data and statistics has been integral to chronicling accounts of injustice against humanity [1]. The connection of surveillance data related to social problems may both expose human exploitation and catapult problems into the public arena provoking a political response [2, 3]. In the case of child labour, data collection and analysis has been paramount in harnessing global action against the use of children in exploitative work.

The purpose of this chapter is to provide an overview of child labour data by a discussion of the historical context of data on children's work; available child labour data definitions; methodologies and sources; global estimates on children's work and some discussion on how data collection will be improved in the near future.

Historical context of child labour data

In 1919, the United Nations founded the International Labour Organization (ILO) to promote social justice, uphold workers' rights, and develop labour standards on working conditions and workplace practices: this included the elimination of child labour [4]. Not until decades later did the enormity of international child labour reach global awareness. In 1993, the ILO's International Programme on the Elimination of Child Labour (IPEC), through its Statistical Information and Monitoring Programme on Child Labour (SIMPOC) together with their Bureau of Statistics, embarked on an ambitious undertaking to design and develop quantitative estimates of the magnitude of child labour. Accurate child labour statistics are essential for establishing targets, formulating interventions, and monitoring the impact of child labour policies, regulations and programmes [5].

The initial phase of the ILO-IPEC's data collection exercise consisted of testing the data estimation methodology by partnering national statistical offices and carrying out experimental surveys in Ghana, India, Indonesia, and Senegal. Subsequently, the methodology was refined and tested in additional countries to estimate the prevalence of child labour at the national level. Together, the results from both rounds of surveys were used to produce the first global estimate on working children [5]. Globally, the ILO estimated that there were 250 million working children in 1995 [6]. The publicity surrounding the new data not only called attention to the magnitude of children working in potentially exploitive and hazardous situations, but also elevated child labour in public awareness and political consciousness [7, 8].

The release of the ILO's 250 million estimate in 1995 was also vital to rallying support for the eventual adoption of ILO Convention No. 182 on the Worst Forms of Child Labour in June 1999. In October 1997, the Government of Norway, together with the ILO and the United Nations Children's Fund (UNICEF), hosted a 40-nation ministerial conference in Oslo to develop an 'Agenda for Action' for the global elimination of child labour. Participants included national ministers representing development, education, labour, social welfare, and justice; employers' organizations; trade union leaders and workers' rights groups; non-governmental organizations; international agencies; and multilateral development banks [9]. Among the principal areas for action, the availability of dependable data was identified as vital for policy, programme development and for advocacy with regard to the elimination of child labour [10]. As a result of this commitment, the ILO, UNICEF, and the World Bank in 2000 formed an interagency research initiative, Understanding Children's Work, to coordinate and standardize data collection and reporting activities on child labour [11].

Child labour data definitions, methodologies, and sources

The ILO global estimates on children's work is defined in terms of 'economic activity' as set forth by the System of National Accounts (SNA) and resolution on employment adopted at the Thirteenth International Conference on Labour Statisticians.

> Economic activity covers all market production (paid work) and certain types of non-market production (unpaid work), including production of goods for own use. Whether paid or unpaid, therefore, the activity or occupation could be pursued in either the formal or informal sector and in either urban or rural areas. For example, children in unpaid activities in a market-oriented establishment operated by a relative living in the same household are considered as working in an economic activity. Also, children working as maids or domestic workers in someone else's household are also considered economically active. However, children engaged in domestic chores within their own households are not classified as economically active [8].

In order for a child to be classified as economically active, the child must have performed at least 1 hour of work during a reference week. While the definition of economic activity in the SNA includes individuals seeking work and those who are currently unemployed, the ILO excludes these groups in measuring children's work [8].

ILO data are generally collected on children aged 5–17 years while SIMPOC works with the national statistical offices in each country to determine their desired age cut-offs for reporting on children's work. ILO-IPEC typically classifies data into three categories: *economically active children*, *child labour*, and *children in hazardous work*.

Economically active children or *working children* is the broadest category that includes all children involved in at least 1 hour of economic activity during a reference week. *Child labour* is a narrower subset of economic activity and includes children below 15 years working in violation of international standards, specifically in regards to ILO Convention No. 138 on Minimum Age.

Children in hazardous work represents any child less than 18 years working in hazardous conditions, which may include children working in mining and construction; working with heavy machinery; exposed to pesticides; and children under 18 years working 43 hours or more a week. No universal method for measuring hazardous work for children exists and the ILO relies on national classifications of hazardous work for children and on ILO Recommendation No. 190 accompanying ILO Convention No. 182 on the Worst Forms of Child Labour [12].

Since the 1997 Oslo Agenda for Action, new data collection methodologies have been developed; data sources have become more numerous; and sampling and extrapolation procedures for national and global estimates on child labour have been and continue to be refined. Data collection methodologies on child labour have included qualitative, quantitative, and mixed-methods approaches. Specific methodologies on child labour have taken the form of household-based surveys, baseline studies, establishment/workplace surveys, rapid assessments, street children inquiries, school-based surveys, and community-level inquiries [13–16]. The ILO and UNICEF jointly developed the rapid assessment methodology to investigate the worst forms of child labour, including some of the more hidden and illicit sectors of work, such as commercial sexual exploitation and drug trafficking [17, 18].

The main data sources for national level estimates on children's work are collected through household surveys from ILO-IPEC's SIMPOC, UNICEF's Multiple Indicator Cluster Survey, and the World Bank's Living Standards Measurement Survey.[1] Among the three data sources, SIMPOC surveys are solely focused on measuring children's work and collect detailed information on industry and occupation, including occupational safety and health items. Data collected on workplace exposures and job characteristics include adult supervision; use of personal protective equipment; night work; heavy physical work; job stress; boredom with work; use of tools/equipment; and exposure to chemicals, physical hazards, and biological hazards [19].

Since the establishment of ILO-IPEC's SIMPOC in 1998, more than 60 countries have received technical assistance to attach modules to existing household surveys or carry out stand-alone surveys to collect data on child labour. To date, SIMPOC has assisted with at least 70 national household surveys on child labour.

UNICEF's Multiple Indicator Cluster Survey (MICS) programme began in 1995 and collects data on a variety of child-related indicators, including child labour as

[1] For a more detailed discussion on the differences in these survey programs and limitations of household surveys in terms of collecting data on child labour, refer to Ritualo, Castro, and Gormly [15].

it relates to child protection. In three rounds of MICS surveys (1995, 2000, and 2005/2006), at least 200 surveys have been implemented in 100 countries. In 2009–2010, UNICEF will conduct another round of surveys (MICS4) [20, 21]. The United States Agency for International Development's (USAID) Demographic and Health Surveys (DHS) has also used selected questions from the Multiple Indicator Cluster Survey to produce data on child labour. Data are collected on children 5–14 years old. UNICEF measures child labour in terms of a child's age; hours of work; and type of work, which includes economic activity and domestic work [22, 23]. UNICEF includes children's domestic work within their own households when measuring child labour, so estimates from UNICEF are likely to be higher than those reported from the ILO.

The World Bank's Living Standards Measurement Survey was launched in 1980 to collect and analyse policy-relevant data on social and economic indicators from household surveys. Since 1985, there have been around 50 national surveys in 23 countries that have collected data on child labour [24, 25]. Living Standards Measurement Surveys do not have a standardized age range for which data are collected on children. Like the ILO, the World Bank measures child labour in terms of economic activity.

Table 2.1 summarizes the different data definitions and sources employed to measure child labour. Given the differences in how children's work is defined and variations in survey methodology, it is important to exercise caution when comparing data across countries. Understanding Children's Work has attempted to reconcile these differences by standardizing data across the various sources in terms of economic activity. It also notes that this approach defers making difficult decisions in defining child labour and "drawing a statistical line between acceptable forms of work, on the one hand, and harmful forms that need to be eliminated, on the other" [26]. Understanding Children's Work data have been used to calculate economic activity rates for children in approximately 80 countries (see Appendix A). Data on children's work are available for 5–14 year olds in 54 countries.

Global estimates of children's work

Since the release of the 1995 global estimate of working children, the ILO has provided the most authoritative statistics on children's involvement in the labour force.[2] New global estimates of child labour for 2000 and 2004 were

[2] In UNICEF's 2007 publication, *Progress for Children: A World Fit for Children, Statistical Review*, there were 14% of children 5–14 years, or 158 million, estimated child labourers. The estimate is based on an analysis of UNICEF's database containing MICS and DHS data collected from 1999 to 2006 in 98 countries.

Table 2.1 Data definitions and sources used to measure child labour

Data source	Indicator	Definition	Surveys
ILO	Economically active children/ working children	5–17 years: at least 1 hour of economic work per week	SIMPOC
	Child labour	5–14 years: at least 1 hour of economic work per week	
	Children in hazardous work	5–17 years: at least 1 hour of economic work per week in occupations deemed hazardous, including children working in mining and construction; working with heavy machinery; exposed to pesticides; or working 43 hours or more a week	
UNICEF	Child labour	5–11 years: at least 1 hour of economic work or 28 hours of domestic chores within own household per week 12–14 years: at least 14 hours of economic work or 28 hours of domestic chores within own household per week 15–17 years: at least 43 hours of economic or domestic chores within own household per week	MICS DHS
World Bank	Economically active	Age various across countries: at least 1 hour of economic work per week	LSMS
Understanding Children's Work Project	Economically active children/ working children	5–14 years: at least 1 hour of economic work per week	SIMPOC, MICS, DHS, LSMS, other household surveys

Survey acronyms: MICS – Multiple Indicator Cluster Survey, SIMPOC – Statistical Information and Monitoring Programme on Child Labour, MICS – Multiple Indicator Cluster Survey, DHS – Demographic and Health Surveys, LSMS – Living Standards Measurement Study Surveys

published in the ILO's Global Reports on Child Labour in the follow-up to the ILO Declaration on Fundamental Principles and Rights at Work [6, 27].[3] The availability of data for 2000 and 2004 allowed for the first time a 'trend' analysis

[3] The data presented in these reports were based on the definition of *economic activity*. In 2010, the ILO will be publishing another Global Report on Child Labour under the Follow-up to the ILO Declaration on Fundamental Principles and Rights at Work, and will be issuing global estimates based on the definition of *children in productive activities.*

of child labour prevalence at the global and regional levels, which is presented in the ILO's 2006 Global Report on Child Labour and Global Child Labour Trends: 2000 to 2004 [12].[4]

It is important to note that the global estimates presented in this overview do not include children in unconditional worst forms of child labour or worst forms of child labour other than those in hazardous work. Therefore it does not include children who have been trafficked or are in armed conflict, forced or bonded labour; prostitution or pornography; or other illicit work activities, such as drug trafficking. The ILO attempted to calculate the number of these children with the 2000 data, and produced an estimate of 8.4 million children involved in worst forms of child labour other than hazardous work. However, the 2004 data did not allow for making extrapolations on this category of children.

Figure 2.1 maps a global picture of working children of age 5–14 years using Understanding Children's Work available estimates from various survey years. The blue dots represent countries where data are available for children of other ages. It can be seen that many of the countries with a high prevalence of working children are in Africa. While percentages of children's work provide a useful indicator relative to a country's population, it is also important to consider the absolute numbers of children working in a particular country.

Figure 2.2 maps the absolute number of working children. This map demonstrates how low prevalence rates do not necessarily equate with the largest numbers of working children. For example, although the prevalence of children working in India is low with 4.1% of children 5–14 years working in 2000, India, because of its population size, still has the largest number of working children in the world; approximately 13 million children of age 5–14 years worked in 2000.

Both data maps also illustrate the need for more data collection on child labour. While almost all the countries in Latin America and a majority of African countries have data on children's work, countries in Asia, such as China, Indonesia, Thailand, and Vietnam, still lack data on children's work.

Figure 2.3 presents results published in the ILO's 2006 Global Report on Child Labour entitled 'The End of Child Labour: Within Reach'. The report received wide media coverage with reported significant decreases between 2000 and 2004 in the estimated number of economically active children, child labourers, and children involved in hazardous work. Overall, there were

[4] Due to different statistical procedures and definitions applied to estimating child labour, the global estimates for 2000 and 2004 are not comparable to the global estimate produced in 1995.

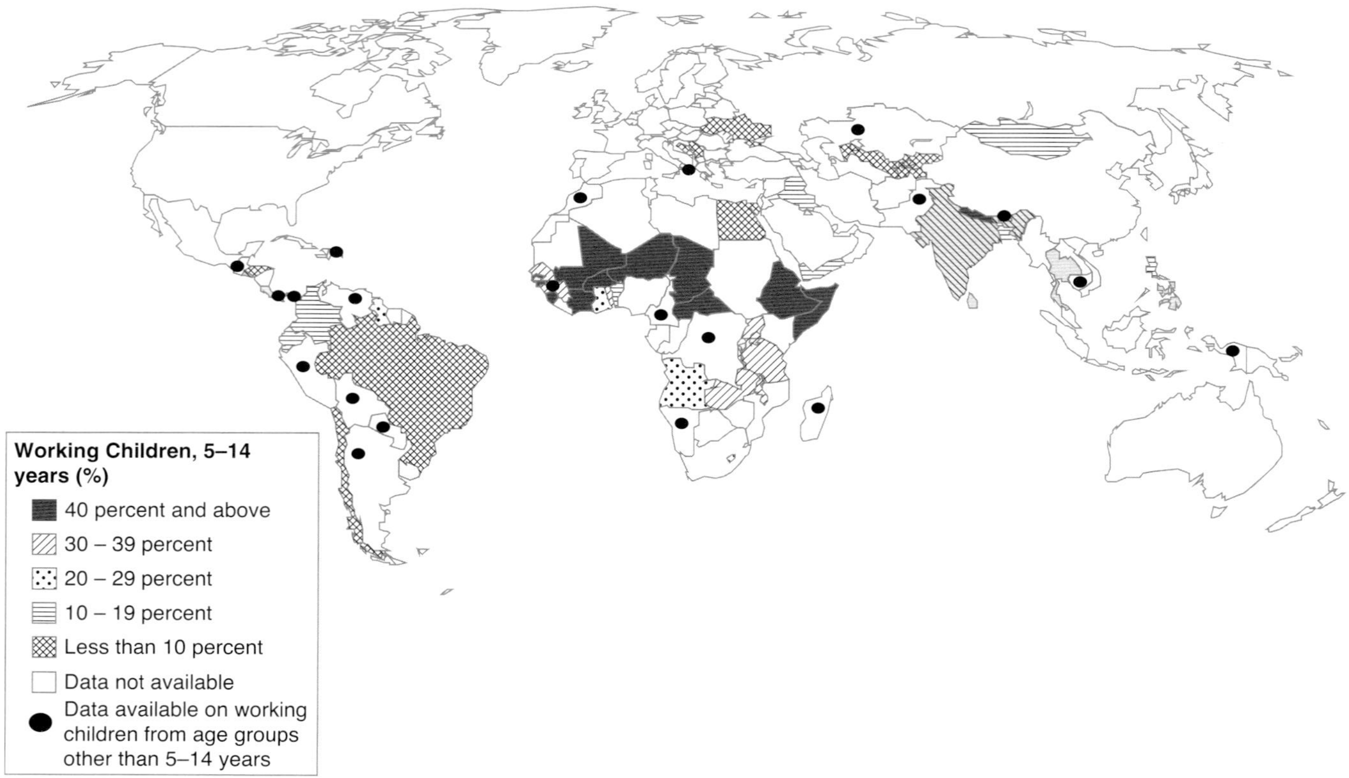

Fig. 2.1 Data availability and percentages of working children, 5–14 years (see inside front cover for colour version).
Source: Author mapping of data from Understanding Children's Work Project's analysis of country statistics from national household or child labour surveys, www.ucw-project.org.

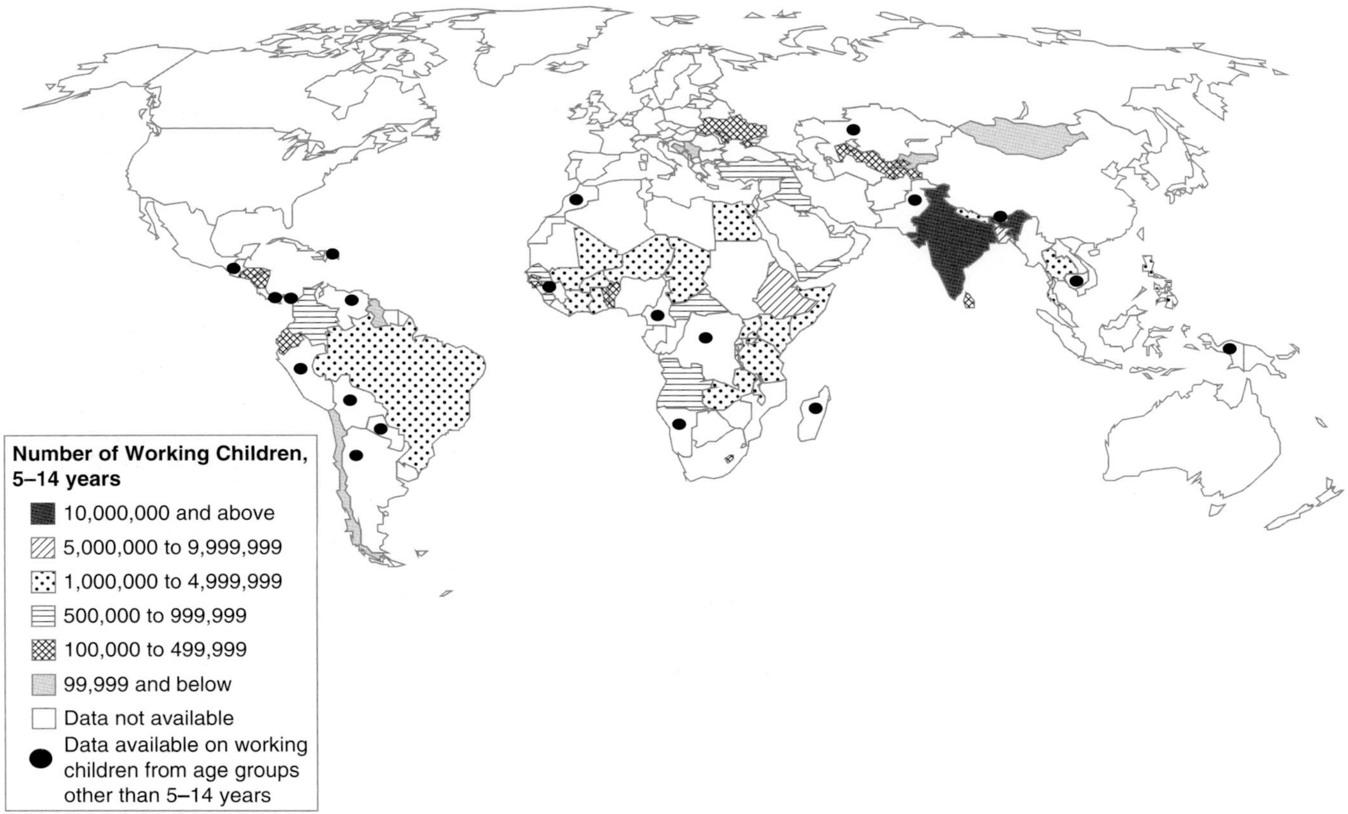

Fig. 2.2 Data availability and absolute numbers of working children, 5–14 years (see inside back cover for colour version).
Source: Author mapping of data from Understanding Children's Work Project's analysis of country statistics from national household or child labour surveys, www.ucw-project.org.

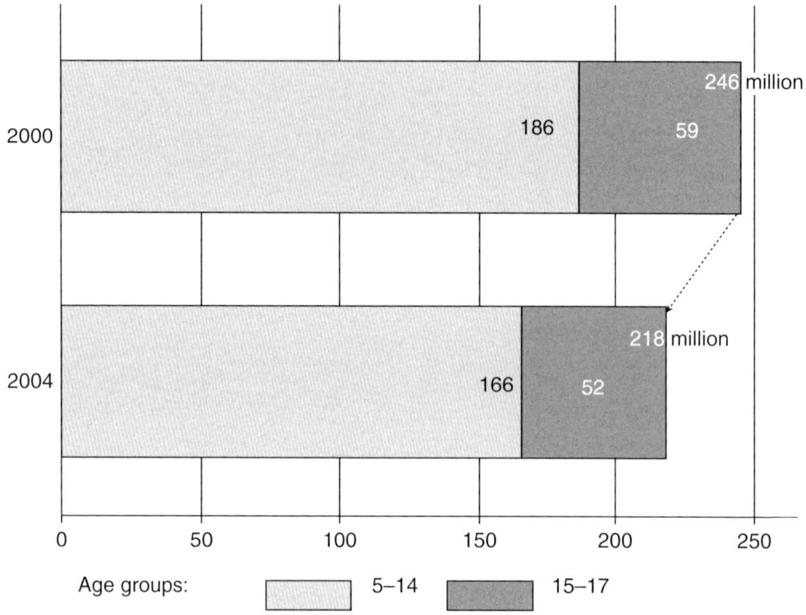

Fig. 2.3 Global trend in the number of child labourers by age group 5–17 years, 2000 and 2004.
Source: ILO, 2006.

317 million working children aged 5–17 years in 2004, 172 million boys compared with 146 million girls. From 2000 to 2004, there was an 11% global decline in the number of child labourers aged 5–17 years (from 246 million in 2000 to 218 million in 2004). For child labourers aged 5–14 years the decrease was 10.8% while among child labourers aged 15–17 years it was 11.9%. This represents 28 million fewer child labourers aged 5–17 years. The largest reduction occurred in children engaged in hazardous work. Even with this decrease, however, the figures still represent an enormous number of children exposed to abuse and exploitation [27].

Table 2.2 presents the regional distribution of working children 5–14 years for 2000 and 2004. Asia and the Pacific continue to represent the region with the largest proportion of working children (64.1%) followed by sub-Saharan Africa (25.9 %). With significant government efforts to tackle the problem of child labour in the 1990s, Latin America shows the greatest decline in working children. Between 2000 and 2004, Latin America witnessed a 67% decline in the numbers of working children. Sub-Saharan Africa is the only region that saw an increase in the number of working children. Figure 2.4 demonstrates that Africa is the region with the highest prevalence of working children compared to all other regions. As discussed later in this book, the impact of

Table 2.2 Regional distribution of working children 5–14 years, 2000 and 2004

Work category	2000		2004		Percent change in numbers of working children
	Number of working children (in millions)	Percent of working children	Number of working children (in millions)	Percent of working children	
Economically active children, 5–14 years	**211.0**	**100.0**	**190.7**	**100.0**	**−9.6**
Region					
Asia and the Pacific	127.3	60.3	122.3	64.1	−3.9
Latin America and the Caribbean	17.4	8.2	5.7	3.0	−67.2
Sub-Saharan Africa	48.0	22.7	49.3	25.9	2.7
Other regions	18.3	8.7	13.4	7.0	−26.8

Source: Hagemann, Diallo, Etienne, and Mehran [12].

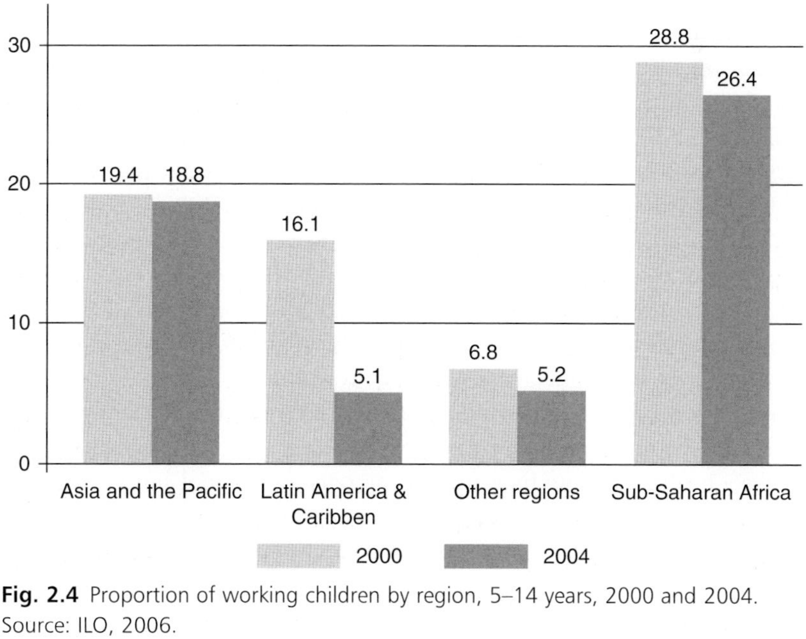

Fig. 2.4 Proportion of working children by region, 5–14 years, 2000 and 2004. Source: ILO, 2006.

HIV/AIDS combined with rising food shortages in Africa, leaves many children vulnerable to early entry into the labour force.

Among working children 5–14 years, children are mainly found working in agriculture, hunting, forestry, and fishing (69%), followed by the services sector (22%) and the industrial sector (9%). In a recent analysis of national surveys conducted from 1999 to 2007 in 15 countries, SIMPOC found that while there were variations in the proportion of working children in agriculture, both boys and girls were involved in agricultural work (see Figure 2.5).

In ILO's 2009 World Day Against Child Labour report entitled, 'Give Girls a Chance: Tackling Child Labour, A Key to the Future', new statistics were released to highlight the vulnerability of girls in the labour force [28]. Of particular concern is the overwhelming representation of girls engaged in domestic work (see Figure 2.6). The hidden nature of girls working in third-party households makes them highly vulnerable to physical abuse and sexual exploitation.

A major data gap in global estimates related to children's work relates to statistics on health indicators. While work-related injuries and illnesses are important indicators of job safety, the latest available statistics are dated and limited. In a 1997 analysis of data from child labour surveys conducted in 26 developing countries, the ILO estimated that 69% of working children are exposed to some kind of work-related hazard. In addition, 70% of reported work-related injuries or illnesses (75.8% in boys and 57.2% in girls) occurred in children working in agriculture [6].

Despite the relative lack of statistics on the health outcomes of working children, the ILO-IPEC's SIMPOC surveys still provide potentially rich data for assessing the relationship between children's work and health outcomes. Using the 2001 Philippine SIMPOC-sponsored survey, Castro, Ritualo, and Gormly [19] detail survey questions used and propose a methodology to assess the risk of injuries and illnesses to working children. Gormly and Ritualo [29] analysed data from the Guatemala, Honduras, and Nicaragua SIMPOC surveys, and presented person-hour incidence rates by age and sex, and described the types of work-related exposures and outcomes. For example, in Nicaragua, 85% of work-related injuries to children involved wounds or cuts, fractures, and bruises. However, long-term outcome data are not available.

In addition, one of Understanding Children's Work core indicators on children's activity measures the percentage of children aged 5–14 years that experience a health problem by economic activity and school status. A health problem is defined as the occurrence of a reported work-related illness or injury. Table 2.3 displays the results of SIMPOC-sponsored surveys in nine countries. It can be seen that in the majority of countries, adverse health outcomes are more likely in children who only work compared to children who combine work with school.

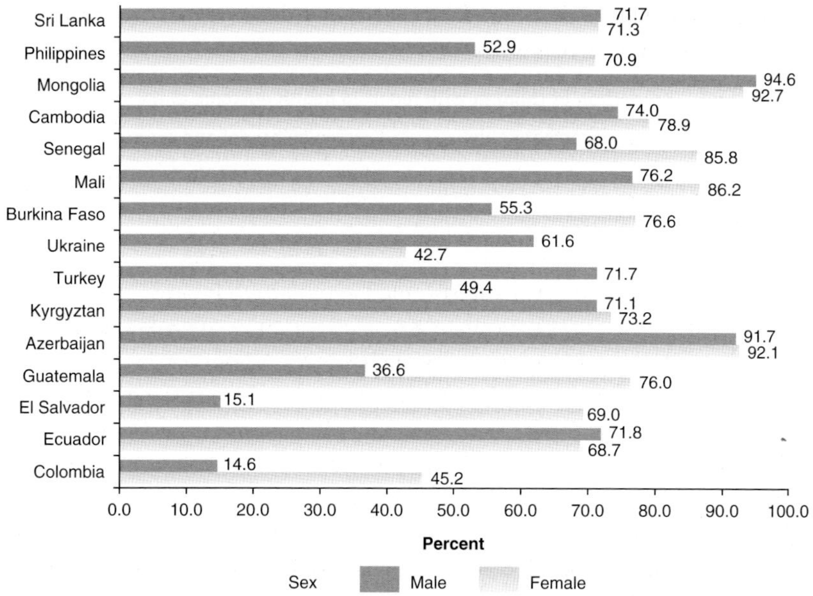

Fig. 2.5 Proportion of working children in agriculture by country and sex, 5–14 years.
Source: SIMPOC calculations of national-level child labour statistics from 15 sample countries.

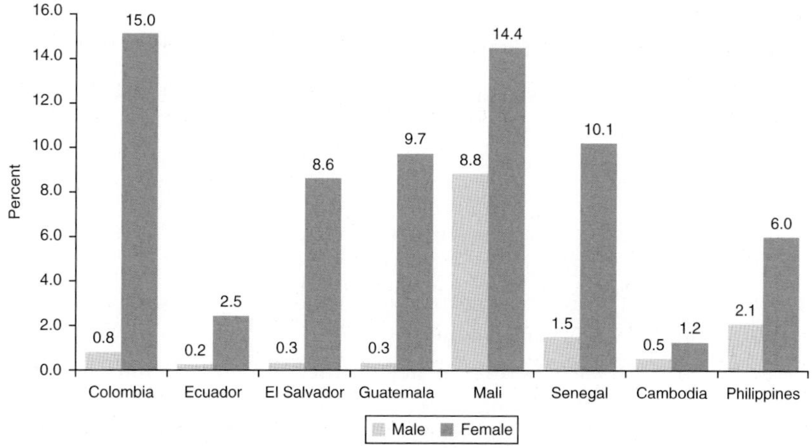

Fig. 2.6 Proportion of working children in domestic work by country and sex, 5–14 years.
Source: SIMPOC calculations of national-level child labour statistics from eight sample countries.

Table 2.3 Percentage of children 5–14 years with reported health outcome by activity status and sex in selected countries

Country and year of survey	Proportion of children with reported health outcome, 5–14 years (in %)					
	Economic activity only			Combining school and economic activity		
	Male	Female	Total	Male	Female	Total
Bangladesh, 2002–2003	11.6	3.1	9.1	2.4	2.4	2.4
Belize, 2001	50.0	33.3	43.2	40.1	22.6	34.0
Cambodia, 2001	57.1	53.1	55.0	48.9	45.6	47.3
Ghana, 2000	30.0	23.3	26.8	31.5	23.5	27.7
Honduras, 2002	17.2	11.2	16.2	9.6	10.8	10.0
Kenya, 1998–1999	17.4	20.1	18.7	28.2	33.2	30.4
Philippines, 2001	40.0	29.5	37.8	27.1	21.8	25.0
Uganda, 2002–2003	9.5	6.8	8.5	8.5	4.8	6.8
Zambia, 1999	5.2	2.3	3.8	2.5	5.3	4.0

Source: Understanding Children's Work Project, Analysis of country statistics from national household or child labour surveys by health indicator and child activity, www.ucw-project.org

Future improvements in child labour data collection

A recent development in statistical measurement and definitions related to children's work can be found in the landmark Resolution Concerning Statistics of Child Labour, adopted on 5 December 2008 at the 18th International Conference of Labour Statisticians (ICLS). Much in the same way the adoption of ILO Convention No. 182 rallied international consensus for the eradication of work that was harmful to children [30], so too was the process for garnering support and negotiating language for agreed child labour statistics. In crafting the resolution, SIMPOC and the Bureau of Statistics consulted with a broad range of partners, such as interagency partners on child labour statistics (UNICEF, World Bank); technical specialists for measuring children's hazardous work; and most importantly, government representatives from both developing and industrialized national statistical offices. One of the most significant outcomes of this resolution is the transition from measuring children's work in terms economic activity to children in productive activities.

This change is important for several reasons. First, using economic activity to measure children's work was deemed erroneous for several reasons. Economic activity was a term developed for measuring adult employment, which includes individuals who are unemployed or seeking work. Therefore, the notion that children should not be looking for work is inconsistent with the definition of economic activity. Children working within the System of National Accounts production boundary for at least an hour are now referred to as 'children in employment'. Second, children performing 'household chores' within their own homes can now be counted as child labour so as long as this work is considered hazardous. This category of children is referred to as 'children in other productive activities or unpaid household services'. Therefore, children in productive activities include children in employment and children in other productive activities [31].

From a gender perspective, this modification to measuring children's work is an acknowledgement of the differences in work carried out by boys and girls, and how the previous approach to measuring children's work underestimated the work of children, primarily girls, in household chores [28, 31].

Conclusions

The growth and development of statistical data collection on child labour has had many positive results, it has at last become possible to accurately monitor trends in child labour and the impact of policies and programmes to address child labour. Perhaps more importantly, the publication of accurate child labour statistics has assisted greatly in harnessing public and political support to reduce the negative consequences of children working.

Despite much effort to harmonize methodologies, different datasets – each established with a slightly different purpose, still exist and there remains some potential for confusion. From the available data it is clear that the prevalence of working children is highest in sub-Saharan Africa although the overall numbers are far greater in Asia. There are still many countries that are likely to have significant numbers of children working, but that do not have accurate data on child labour.

There are a number of improvements that could be made to data collection at little cost. There is a relative lack to of data on the health outcomes from working. National household surveys remain important tools for collecting data on child labour. Occupational health and safety questions should be included in order to capture appropriate data. These could include the average number of hours a child works in a given year (i.e., average days, weeks, and months); the number of injuries that occurred during the reference period; information about the most recent injury event; and the severity of most recent injury event, including work-time restrictions and disability outcomes. These questions would allow both exposure time and health outcomes to be measured.

Many countries have struggled to construct hazardous child labour lists in line with Convention 182. The ILO should encourage member countries to systematically identify hazardous work activities based on empirical evidence. While there are various ways to determine hazardous work activities for children, analysing data from national household surveys would be a cost-effective first step to creating a hazardous list that is nationally representative of the industries and sectors children are engaged in. For countries with limited resources, this method could also assist in focusing attention on the most hazardous industries that deserve immediate attention for prevention efforts. Beyond the data collected from national child labour surveys, qualitative studies through rapid assessments on smaller samples could be conducted in order to further investigate hazardous occupations and processes.

Statistics have a critical role to play in advancing research on child labour. The ability to statistically measure and identify hazardous work for children—both outcome and severity—will do much to advance targeted interventions for the elimination of the worst forms of child labour, and will help set the stage for wider and better efforts to prevent child labour.

Acknowledgements

The author would like to extend appreciation to her colleagues at ILO-IPEC's SIMPOC programme and the Understanding Children's Work project for their dedication to advancing the knowledge base on child labour through data and statistics. Special recognition is owed to Furio Rosati and Lorenzo Guarcello for their timely responses to my numerous data inquiries. The author is extremely grateful to Amy Ritualo and Sarah Gormly Donovan for their earlier work together that formed the foundation for this chapter. Finally, the author would like to recognize Laura Gauer Bermudez and Sarah Newsome for their research assistance.

References

1 Asher J, Banks D, Scheuren FJ (eds) (2008). Statistical methods for Human Rights. New York: Springer.

2 Stone D (1997). Numbers. In: *Policy Paradox: The Art of Political Decision Making*. New York: W. W. Norton & Company, Inc.

3 Kingdon JW (1995). *Agendas, alternatives, and public policies*. Second ed. New York: Longman.

4 International Labour Organization (2004). The ILO: What it is, what it does [Brochure]. Geneva: International Labour Organization.

5 International Labour Office (1996a). Child labour surveys: Results of methodological experiments in four countries 1992–93. Geneva: International Labour Organization.
6 Ashagrie K (1998). Statistics on working children and hazardous child labour in brief. Geneva: International Labour Office.
7 International Labour Office (1996b). Child labour: targeting the intolerable. Geneva: International Labour Organization.
8 International Labour Office (2002). Every child counts: new global estimates on child labour. Geneva: International Labour Office.
9 International Labour Organization (1997). International Conference on Child Labour Oslo, 27–30 October 1997. Geneva: International Labour Organization.
10 International Labour Organization (1997). Oslo conference to seek global strategy for combating child labour. Geneva: International Labour Organization.
11 Understanding Children's Work Project (2001). The Understanding Children's Work (UCW) Project: A Research Initiative of the International Labour Organization, UNICEF and the World Bank [Brochure]. Rome: UCW Project Secretariat.
12 Hagemann F, Diallo Y, Etienne A, Mehran F (2006). Global child labour trends: 2000 to 2004. Geneva: International Labour Office.
13 International Labour Office (2004). Child labour statistics: manual on methodologies for data collection through surveys. Geneva: International Labour Organization.
14 International Labour Office (2008). Report III, child labour statistics. Geneva: International Labour Organization.
15 Ritualo AR, Castro CL, Gormly S (2003). Measuring child labor: Implications for policy and program design. *Comparative Labor Law and Policy Journal*, **24**(2):401–34.
16 Verma V (2008). Sampling for household-based surveys of child labour. Geneva: International Labour Organization.
17 International Labour Organization, UNICEF (2000). Investigating child labour: Guidelines for rapid assessment, a field manual. Geneva: ILO and UNICEF.
18 International Labour Office (2005). Investigating the worst forms of child labour: A synthesis report of selected rapid assessment and national reports. Geneva: International Labour Organization.
19 Castro CL, Gormly S, Ritualo AR (2005). The SIMPOC Philippine survey of children 2001: A data source for analyzing occupational injuries to children. *Public Health Reports*, **120**(6):631–41.
20 UNICEF. Statistics and monitoring: Multiple Indicator Cluster Surveys (MICS) (n.d.) http://www.unicef.org/statistics/index_24302.html
21 UNICEF. Multiple Indicator Cluster Surveys (MICS) (2009). http://www.unicef.org/statistics/index_24302.html
22 UNICEF (2007). Progress for children: A world fit for children statistical review. New York: UNICEF. http://www.unicef.org/statistics/index_24302.html
23 UNICEF. Statistics by Area/Child Protection (2009).
24 Grosh M, Glewwe P (1995). a guide to living standards measurement study surveys and their data sets, LSMS Working Paper no. 120. Washington, DC: The World Bank.
25 The World Bank. Living Standards Measurement Study (n.d.) The World Bank. http://www.childinfo.org/protection.html

26 Cigno A, Guarcello L, Noguchi Y, Lyon S, Rosati F (2003). Child labour indicators used by the UCW project: An explanatory note. Rome: Understanding Children's Work Project. http://econ.worldbank.org/WBSITE/EXTERNAL/EXTDEC/EXTRESEARCH/EXTLSMS/0,,contentMDK:21478196~menuPK:3359066~pagePK:64168445~piPK:64168309~theSitePK:3358997,00.html

27 International Labour Office (2006). The end of child labour: Within reach, Global Report under the Follow-up to the ILO Declaration on Fundamental Principles and Rights at Work. Geneva: International Labour Office.

28 International Labour Office (2009). Give girls a chance: Tackling child labour, a key to the future. Geneva: International Labour Office.

29 Gormly S, Ritualo AR (2005). When is child work hazardous? Evidence from the SIMPOC surveys. Washington, DC. http://paa2005.princeton.edu/abstractViewer.aspx?submissionId=51717

30 Myers WE (2001). The right rights? *Annals of the American Academy of Political and Social Science*, **575**(1):38–55.

31 International Labour Organization (2008). Resolution concerning statistics of child labour, Adopted by the Eighteenth International Conference of Labour Statisticians. Geneva: International Labour Organization.

Appendix A

Table 2.1 Data availability on working children

Country	Year	Age range (years)	Survey source	Child population			Working children (in %)		
				Total	Male	Female	Total	Male	Female
Afghanistan									
Albania	2000	7–14	MICS	567,247	290,033	277,214	36.6	41.1	31.8
Algeria									
Angola	2001	5–14	MICS	2,415,041	1,198,709	1,216,332	25.7	25.6	25.9
Anguilla									
Argentina	1997	10–14	WB	2,858,933	1,444,135	1,414,798	20.7*	25.4	16.0
Armenia									
Bahrain									
Bangladesh	2006	5–14	MICS3	37,340,058	18,971,013	18,369,046	13.6	21.3	5.6
Barbados									
Belize	2001	5–14	SIMPOC	63,350	31,704	31,646	6.3	8.1	4.6
Benin	2002–03	5–14	LSMS	2,086,870	1,129,888	956,982	13.2	11.5	15.3
Bhutan	2003	10–14	LSMS	73,671	34,576	39,095	19.6	16.1	22.7
Bolivia	2002	7–14	HHS	1,783,061	932,633	850,428	23.2	23.9	22.5
Bosnia and Herzegovina	2006	5–14	MICS3	496,613	246,926	249,686	8.9	9.9	7.9

(Continued)

Table 2.1 (continued) Data availability on working children

Country	Year	Age range (years)	Survey source	Child population			Working children (in %)		
				Total	Male	Female	Total	Male	Female
Botswana									
Brazil	2004	5–14	PNAD	34,367,074	17,502,567	16,864,507	5.2	7.0	3.3
British Indian Ocean Territory									
British Virgin Islands									
Burkina Faso	2003	5–14	HHS	3,462,184	1,780,136	1,682,047	47.0	46.4	47.7
Burundi	2000	5–14	MICS	2,162,500	1,034,792	1,127,708	31.2	32.3	30.1
Cambodia	2003–04	10–14	HHS	1,817,863	924,885	892,978	48.9	49.6	48.1
Cameroon	2001	10–14	LSMS	2,056,541	1,045,563	1,010,978	15.9	14.5	17.4
Cape Verde	2001–02	10–14	HHS	142,407	72,871	69,536	3.2	3.8	2.6
Central African Republic	2000	5–14	MICS	1,330,919	669,383	661,536	61.1	60.4	61.7
Chad	2004	5–14	DHS	2,898,858	1,469,866	1,428,992	53.0	56.1	49.7
Chad	2000	5–14	MICS	2,493,116	1,235,632	1,257,484	62.7	65.3	60.0
Chile	2003	5–14	SIMPOC	2,800,255	1,437,555	1,362,700	3.5	4.4	2.6

Christmas Island									
Cocos Islands									
Colombia	2001	5–14	SIMPOC	8,580,980	4,358,012	4,222,967	10.4	14.1	6.6
Colombia	1998	10–14	LSMS	4,205,064	2,079,775	2,125,289	8.0	11.9	4.1
Comoros	2000	5–14	MICS	159,810	82,560	77,250	35.6	35.0	36.2
Congo									
Cook Islands									
Costa Rica	2004	12–14	HHS	264,993	126819	138174	5.7	8.1	3.5
Cote d'Ivoire	2006	5–14	MICS3	5,478,424	2822505	2655919	39.8	41.5	38.0
Croatia									
Democratic Republic of the Congo	2000	10–14	MICS	7,098,056	3,502,322	3,595,734	39.8	39.9	39.8
Djibouti									
Dominica									
Dominican Republic	2005	10–14	LFS	1035151	510760	524391	5.8	9.0	2.7
East Timor	2001	10–14	LSMS	100,087	51,980	48,107	85.2	84.5	85.9
Ecuador	2004	5–14	SIMPOC	2,969,088	1,507,999	1,461,089	10.2	12.6	7.8
Egypt	2005	5–14	DHS	15,247,673	7,809,925	7,437,747	6.7	9.5	3.7
El Salvador	2003	5–14	SIMPOC	1,598,487	785,144	813,343	10.2	13.7	6.5
Equatorial Guinea									

(Continued)

Table 2.1 (continued) Data availability on working children

Country	Year	Age range (years)	Survey source	Child population			Working children (in %)		
				Total	Male	Female	Total	Male	Female
Eritrea									
Ethiopia	2005	5–14	LFS	17,722,972	9,103,073	8,619,899	50.1	58.1	41.6
Ethiopia	99/00	10–14	LSMS	7,463,159	3,755,462	3,707,697	4.0	5.8	2.2
Falkland Islands									
Fiji									
Gabon									
Gambia	2005–06	5–14	MICS3	496918	239666	257252	36.4	28.5	43.8
Georgia									
Ghana	2000	5–14	SIMPOC	5,174,923	2,689,340	2,485,583	24.2	24.5	24.0
Gibraltar									
Grenada									
Guatemala	2003	7–14	LFS	2550744	1273897	1276847	21.1	26.2	16.0
Guinea	1994	7–14	LSMS	1,477,357	790,439	686,918	48.8*	47.6*	50.2*
Guinea Bissau	2000	5–14	MICS	385,726	195,734	189,992	64.2	64.4	64.0
Guyana	2000	5–14	MICS	172,342	86,291	86,051	26.3	28.7	23.9
Haiti	2005	5–14	DHS	2,271,815	1,130,530	1,141,285	29.0	32.2	26.0
Heard Island and McDonald Islands									

Honduras	2004	5–14	HHS	1,941,242	971,668	969,574	5.4	8.2	2.6
India	1999/2000	5–14	HHS	311,864,479	165,109,977	146,754,502	4.1	4.1	4.0
Indonesia			UCW						
Iraq	2006	5–14	MICS3	7,074,168	3,602,455	3,471,712	12.4	15.1	9.6
Jamaica	2006	5–14	MICS3	573192	292392	280801	8.4	9.6	7.2
Jordan									
Kazakhstan	1996	7–14	LSMS	3,023,475	1,585,675	1,437,800	29.7	30.3	29.1
Kenya	2000	5–14	MICS	9,047,128	4,516,608	4,530,520	32.5	34.7	30.4
Kiribati									
Kyrgyzstan	2006	5–14	MICS3	1,075,630	542,902	532,729	4.5	5.1	3.9
Lebanon									
Lesotho	2000	5–14	MICS	443,297	220,983	222,314	28.1	31.3	25.0
Liberia									
Madagascar	2001	6–14	LSMS	3,782,808	1,910,457	1,872,351	24.3	24.8	23.7
Malawi	2004	5–14	DHS	3,657,292	1,791,873	1,865,419	35.9	38.0	34.0
Mali	2005	5–14	SIMPOC	3,664,237	1,886,076	1,778,162	65.8	66.6	64.9
Mauritania									
Mauritius									
Mongolia	2005	5–14	MICS3	571,782	287,983	283,799	11.3	12.9	9.8
Montserrat									
Morocco	98/99	7–14	LSMS	5,226,523	2,681,411	2,545,112	13.2	13.5	12.8

(Continued)

Table 2.1 (continued) Data availability on working children

Country	Year	Age range (years)	Survey source	Child population			Working children (in %)		
				Total	Male	Female	Total	Male	Female
Mozambique									
Namibia	1999	6–14	SIMPOC	325,394	160,640	164,754	14.7	15.5	13.9
Nepal	1999	5–14	LFS	4,989,490	2,559,353	2,430,137	39.6	35.4	44.0
Nicaragua	2005	5–14	HHS	1,300,494	660,058	640,436	8.4	13.5	3.2
Niger	2000	5–14	MICS	3,140,254	1,560,938	1,579,316	66.2	71.8	60.6
Nigeria									
Niue									
Norfolk Island									
Oman									
Pakistan	1999–2000	10–14	LFS	13,550,151	7,113,697	6,436,454	16.4	15.8	17.2
Panama	2003	10–14	HHS	319,968	166,674	153,294	5.1	7.7	2.2
Papua N. Guinea									
Paraguay	2005	10–14	HHS	739,776	375,096	364,680	15.3	22.6	7.7
Peru	2000	6–14	LSMS	5,420,818	2,785,898	2,634,920	22.3	24.0	20.5
Philippines	2001	5–14	SIMPOC	19,874,678	10,272,020	9,602,658	11.0	13.4	8.4
Pitcairn Islands									
Republic of Moldova	2000	5–14	MICS	712,734	359,628	353,106	30.1	31.2	28.9

Russia									
Rwanda	2000	5–14	MICS	2,497,644	1,210,924	1,286,720	27.3	29.9	24.8
Saint Helena									
Samoa									
Sao Tome & Principe	2000	5–14	MICS	40,435	20,585	19,850	15.4	17.2	13.5
Senegal	2005	5–14	DHS	2,983,310	1,481,658	1,501,652	30.0	33.4	26.7
Seychelles									
Serbia	2005	5–14	MICS3	895,616	460,866	434,751	6.0	6.4	5.7
Montenegro	2005	5–14	MICS3	99,990	52,733	47,256	12.9	14.6	11.0
Sierra Leone	2005	5–14	MICS3	1,670,733	837,834	832,899	58.5	59.0	58.0
Solomon Islands									
Somalia	2006	5–14	MICS3	2,544,081	1,294,018	1,250,063	39.8	41.2	38.4
South Africa									
Sri Lanka	1998	5–14	SIMPOC	3,186,838	1,657,257	1,529,580	15.0	17.9	11.9
St Kitts & Nevis									
St Lucia									
St Vincent and the Grenadines									
Suriname									
Swaziland	2000.0	5–14	MICS	282227.0	143302.0	138925.0	9.6	9.6	9.6

(Continued)

Table 2.1 (continued) Data availability on working children

Country	Year	Age range (years)	Survey source	Child population			Working children (in %)		
				Total	Male	Female	Total	Male	Female
Tajikistan	2005	5–14	MICS3	1,734,940	910,685	824,255	7.3	7.3	7.4
Thailand	2005–06	5–14	MICS3	9990624.0	5112982.0	4877641.0	13.0	13.5	12.6
The Former Yugoslav Rep. of Macedonia									
Togo	2006	5–14	WB	1,461,377	756,684	704,694	32.7	33.7	31.6
Tokelau									
Tonga									
Trinidad and Tobago	2000	5–14	MICS	257,049	126,836	130,213	3.5	4.5	2.6
Tunisia									
Turkey	1999	5–14	SIMPOC	12,065,538	6,154,352	5,911,186	4.2	4.6	3.7
Turks and Caicos Islands									
Tuvalu									
Uganda	2005–2006	5–14	HHS	8,749,882	4,365,814	4,384,068	31.1	32.4	29.8
Ukraine	1999	5–14	SIMPOC	6,933,779	3,538,457	3,395,322	2.4	3.0	1.8
Tanzania	2001	5–14	SIMPOC	9,829,325	4,987,949	4,841,376	35.4	36.2	34.5
Uruguay									

Uzbekistan	2006	5–14	MICS3	5,713,864	2,886,323	2,827,541	4.3	4.4	4.1
Vanuatu									
Venezuela	2005	10–14	HHS	2,753,796	1,405,717	1,348,079	5.4	7.1	3.6
Venezuela	2000	10–14	LSMS	2,669,182	1,361,673	1,307,509	4.8	7.2	2.4
Wallis and Futuna									
West Bank & Gaza Strip									
Western Sahara									
Yemen	1999	5–14	HHS	5,936,728	2,891,301	3,045,427	11.1	11.2	11.0
Zambia	2005	5–14	LFS	3,253,153	1,642,463	1,610,690	33.4	34.4	32.4
Zimbabwe									

Source: Understanding Children's Work Compilation of Data on Working Children

Part 2

A model of child labour

Chapter 3

A rights-oriented, public health model of child labour

Anaclaudia G. Fassa, David L. Parker, and Thomas J. Scanlon

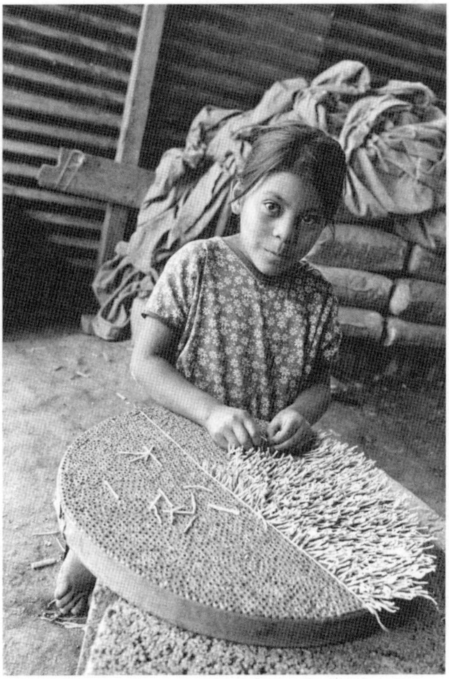

Making fireworks, Guatemala

Introduction

This section introduces the conceptual framework for child labour that underpins subsequent contributions to this volume. The framework is based on a rights-oriented public health approach and the child labour model presented illustrates those principles.

Child work has been defined in terms of economic activity by the Thirteenth International Conference of Labour Statisticians [1]. Economic activity covers all market production (i.e. paid work) and certain types of non-market production (i.e. unpaid work), including the production of goods for a family's own use. Children engaged in domestic chores in their own household are not classified as economically active unless this work means that they are removed from school and/or activities of social development.

Child labour is frequently used as a generic term referring to all work activity of children and adolescents. However, this use fails to distinguish between work that is harmful and work that may contribute to development. The definition of child labour used in the model described below includes 'child labour' and 'hazardous child work' as defined by the ILO[1] and its Statistical Information and Monitoring Programme on Child Labour (SIMPOC). A full discussion of definitions is included in the previous section entitled 'An overview of child labour statistics'.

The rights-oriented public health model of child labour

The harmful impact of child labour is usually considered in terms of the immediate harm to the individual child. There is less attention paid to the impact of work on growth and development and the long-term impact of early work is not always fully considered. The wider impact on the family, and how child labour impacts, or is impacted upon by the community is rarely explored.

Public health has been defined as 'the science and art of preventing disease, prolonging life and promoting health through the organized efforts

---

[1] Not all work done by children should be classified as child labour that is to be targeted for elimination. Children's or adolescents' participation in work that does not affect their health and personal development or interfere with their schooling is generally regarded as being something positive. This includes activities such as helping their parents around the home, assisting in a family business or earning pocket money outside school hours and during school holidays. These kinds of activities contribute to children's development and to the welfare of their families; they provide them with skills and experience, and help to prepare them to be productive members of society during their adult life.

Three groups of working children are identified in ILO figures: (1) Economically-active children/working children refers to children aged 5–17 years who undertake a least 1 hour of economic work per week; (2) Child labour refers to children aged 5–14 years engaged in at least 1 hour of economic work per week; (3) Children in hazardous work refers to children aged 5–17 years engaged in at least 1 hour of economic activity per week in occupations deemed hazardous, including children working in mining and construction, working with heavy machinery, exposed to pesticides; or working 43 hours or more a week.

and informed choices of society, organizations, public and private, communities and individuals' [2]. A public health model offers the potential for a developmental and community-oriented approach that explains child labour in a holistic context, taking into account the wider determinants of child labour, how they interact, and how in turn they are affected by child labour.

The model illustrated in Figure 3.1 shows the domains that comprise the causes and consequences of child labour at the individual, family, and community levels. The five causal domains depicted in the top half of the figure are economics, education, social values, public health and wellbeing, and legislation and its enforcement. Each domain exerts a direct effect on child labour and mediates through the other domains. For example, it is well established that education impacts family health and wellbeing.

The lower half of the model depicts the impact of child labour on the child, family, and community. More immediate effects (hazardous exposures, income) are separated from the longer-term consequences. This separation is not, however, always clear. For example, some health effects such as injuries may have both short- and long-term impact. In addition, short-term consequences in a domain, such as income generation which appear positive,

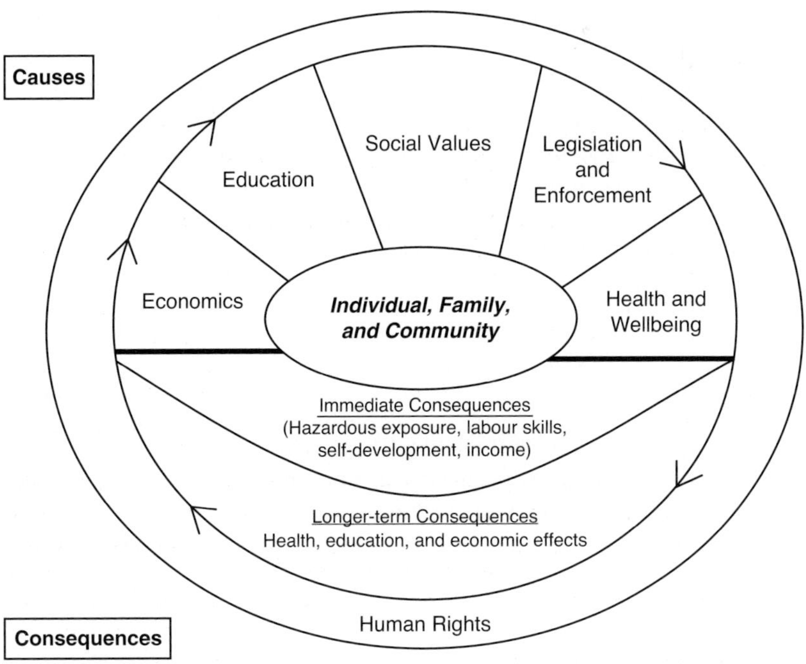

Fig. 3.1 A rights-oriented public health model of child labour.

may in fact have long-term negative consequences such as reduced long-term employment prospects.

The model illustrates the cyclical nature of child labour. The consequences of child labour such as higher rates of illiteracy, compromised health from exposure to hazards, and slowed economic development contribute to a cycle of poor health, low levels of education, and poverty that affects the wider population and sustains a child workforce.

The model as a whole is framed in the context of human rights where every child has the right to be provided for and to be protected and where communities have the right to participate in decisions related to their wellbeing.

The content of this volume in relation to the model

A brief summary of the basis for the selection of the different domains is given below. Each domain is explored more fully within subsequent individual chapters. The other sections of this book and how they relate to the model are also briefly described.

Economics

There is a strong association between economic status and child labour. This association occurs both at the macro-economic and micro-economic (community and family) levels [3]. The income that comes from child labour can be essential to families' short-term survival. However, child work that compromises the health of children and the wider community has long-term adverse consequences for economic development. Interventions which alleviate poverty and invest in human capital play an important role in tackling child labour. In addition to providing benefits to poor families, they can have wider effects on education and on the health status of children and family members in both the short and the long term.

Education

Countries with low school enrolment rates typically have high prevalence rates of child labour. Compulsory primary education has been cited as the key policy instrument by which states can effectively remove children from the labour force [4]. When work hampers education, it diminishes a child's future ability to get a higher quality job and the wages that accompany it. Low levels of education help sustain poverty which in turn pushes children into the workforce in order to guarantee subsistence.

There is a consistent and strong association between a lack of education and poorer long-term health. Thus, an impaired education contributes to a cycle of child labour through poor health as well as impaired income. Educational interventions have the potential for a wide effect including improving public health and wellbeing and economic prosperity [5, 6].

Social values

There is little empirical research on the role of social values in the determination of child labour. However, there is some evidence that the prevalence of child labour is determined by how societies understand and value childhood, work, and education. In some societies, the status of children is related to the amount and type of work they are able to undertake. Communities may have a long heritage of children following their parents' footsteps into traditional occupations. In such situations, undertaking work fulfills societal expectations and is a confirmation of belonging. In some of these cases, work becomes a strong part of a community's identity [7]. Social and cultural values may outweigh the pressures from child labour legislation and attempts to impose such legislation without consideration of these values may prove counter-productive.

Health

There is a lack of good quality studies on the health effects of child labour, and a need for better designed studies. Nevertheless, there are data from child labour-specific studies – many from developed countries, from studies of children exposed to hazards outside of work, and from occupational exposures to adults. With some caveats, these can shed considerable light on the health impact of child labour.

The potential adverse impact of work on the health of children and their communities is considerable. This can occur through premature illness and disability, in the individual as well as in the community through, for example, environmental contamination. Adverse consequences may also be mediated through the interaction of poor health with other determinants of child labour such as education and economic development.

Legislation

International legislation has been at the forefront of addressing child labour since the creation of the ILO in 1919 [8]. There is a wide range of international legislation addressing child labour, much of it focused on children's rights. In recent years, the legislative focus has moved from prohibition and minimum age requirements to the elimination of the worst forms of child labour and the identification and elimination of hazardous child work.

Where individual countries have adopted comprehensive measures to tackle child labour, the enactment and enforcement of national legislation has been important in raising awareness, gaining momentum, and in harnessing high level commitment to change.

Rights

Framing this public health model within the wider context of human rights adds an important dimension. A consequence of this is that interventions to address child labour within each domain cannot be considered without a broader consideration of rights. Interventions must be designed and introduced in a manner that does not compromise rights and actively promotes the rights of children, families, and communities.

The relation of other sections of the volume to the model

The other sections of this volume have been written in the context of the rights-oriented public health model. The overview of child labour statistics previously presented in this book, includes discussion on the importance of data in profiling child labour activity as well as monitoring progress in its control. The policy case studies from Brazil, Kenya, and the Philippines report on how these countries have sought to address child labour, and are described with reference to the domains identified in the model. The main focus of the Brazil case study is economic interventions while the Kenya and the Philippines case studies consider the impact of comprehensive International Programme on Elimination of Child Labour (IPEC) time-bound projects. Three subsequent smaller case studies illustrate particular parts of the model. The Rugmark and the North American Guidelines for Children's Agricultural Task case studies discuss how non-governmental interventions can reduce the adverse impact of children's work in particular settings. The study of coco-babaçu workers in northeast Brazil illustrates how child labour legislation enacted with the rights of children in mind, can conflict with other rights as identified by traditional communities.

Conclusions

The final section of the book contains a discussion on what may be learned from taking a rights-oriented public health approach to child labour based on a full consideration of the contributions from the various authors.

It is the belief of the editors that a rights-oriented public health approach provides a fuller understanding of child labour, its causes, consequences, and its cyclical nature. The proposed model is offered as a mechanism whereby a broader perspective can be taken, where outcomes are clearly defined and evaluated and where more comprehensive, inclusive, and sustainable solutions can be developed.

References

1 International Labour Organisation (ILO) (1982). Resolution concerning statistics of the economically active population, employment, unemployment and underemployment, Thirteenth International Conference of Labour Statisticians. Geneva: ILO.

2 Winslow CEA (1920). The untilled fields of public health. *Science*, 50.

3 Edmonds E (2008). Child labor. In Schultz TP, Strauss J (eds), *Handbook of Development Economics*, Vol. 4, pp. 3607–3710. Amsterdam: Elsevier Science.

4 Weiner M (1991). *The child and the state in India*. Princeton, New Jersey: Princeton University Press.

5 Myers WE (2001). Valuing diverse approaches to child labor. In Lieten K, White B (eds), *Child Labour: Policy Options*. Amsterdam: Aksant.

6 Salazar MC, Glasinovich WA (1996). Better schools: Less child work and education in Brazil, Colombia, Ecuador, Guatemala and Peru. Innocenti Essays no. 7. Florence, Italy: UNICEF International Child Development Centre.

7 Woodhead M (2001). The value of work and school: A study of working children's perspectives. In Lieten K, White B (eds),*Child Labour: Policy Options*. Amsterdam: Aksant.

8 Treaty of Versailles, June 28, 1919, 225 Consol. T.S. 188, 2 Bevans 43.

Chapter 4

Public health in the economics of child labour

Eric V. Edmonds

Introduction

Most of the world's economically active children work by their parents' side, often in a family farm or business. A 2000 UNICEF project surveyed working children in 36 developing countries [1]. The data represent more than 120 million children of ages 5 to14 years. Although nearly 70% of children in these countries spend time in some form of economic activity or domestic chores, less than 3% work in the formal wage labour market [2]. Most of this wage employment, like most employment overall in the world's poorest economies, is in agriculture.

The specific public and personal health concerns associated with child labour will vary from task to task and across working environments. A child in a carpet factory, mine, or brick yard will face different risks from a child in agriculture. Other chapters in this volume consider the health risks associated with different jobs and tasks. These risks influence the private calculation of whether to send a child to work and the public calculation about the costs of that work in very much the same way. This chapter does not distinguish between safety issues, work environment issues, and more general health issues associated with a specific work setting.

Public health is important in the child labour discussion for more reasons than just the consequences of child labour. The morbidity and mortality of caregivers and earners may be central in understanding how children end up in dangerous or exploitive conditions. The purpose of this chapter is to outline how public health issues enter into the economics of child labour. It examines both how public health influences child labour and how child labour influences child health. This chapter begins by reviewing the state of economic research on why children work.

The economics of child labour

Children are more likely to work in poor countries than in rich countries. Nearly three-fourths of the cross-country variation in economic activity rates can be explained by gross domestic product (GDP) per capita alone, and children rarely work in countries with a GDP per capita of US $8,400 or more [3]. Rich and poor countries differ in many ways. This strong cross-country correlation does not necessarily imply a causal relationship, but there is an abundance of evidence that suggests child labour and poverty are closely linked.

Poor families balance the child's potential economic contribution against alternative uses of the child's time. What is the child's potential economic contribution? Direct wage income paid to working children may be important in some contexts, but wage work is rare. In most situations, working children's primary economic contribution comes through the help they offer to their families. Most often, this help is providing domestic services that free up adult time for income-generating pursuits. When there is a family business or farm, the child and other family members often help, and working in the family business or farm is the most prevalent economic activity of children. The value of the child's economic contribution to family farms and businesses can be large. One recent study from Nepal estimates that children are responsible for nearly 9% of the nation's GDP [4].

It should be obvious that the child's potential economic contribution, whether earned as wages or in the form of the child's contribution to household production, depends on the child's local economic environment. Children are better at some tasks than others. Skill-intensive work excludes most children who are not likely to have had the appropriate education or training. Similarly, activities that require strength and physical development tend to be relatively difficult for young children. For example, certain industries in Brazil, such as the cultivation of cotton and tobacco, are more child-intensive than industries such as lumber or root cultivation [5]. Declines in child-intensive industries accounts for around 30% of the decline in child labour in rural Brazil between 1980 and 2000.

The availability of land, livestock, and other productive assets within the household can be an important influence on the child's potential net economic contribution. Children can only work in family businesses when there is one. Given that wage child labour is rare in most countries, studies frequently find that children are more likely to work if their household owns a business. Some types of businesses and productive household assets are more conducive to child involvement than others. For example, children in Ethiopian families are more likely to work on the farm when there is small livestock present rather than large livestock [6]. Of course, families that own productive assets are often wealthier than families without productive assets. A recent study from north India documents that the relationship between family landholdings and child labour follows an inverted U-shape: poor children are more likely to work and to work more intensively as their family adds productive assets, but at some point, child labour declines with the addition of productive assets as the family becomes sufficiently wealthy to avoid child labour [7].

This latter observation from India hints at how important poverty is as a determinant of whether children work. During an economic crisis, when the child's potential economic contribution declines, researchers often find that children work more. For example, one recently documented study found that children transition in and out of employment in reaction to adult unemployment spells in urban Brazil [8]. Another study observes that children work more when coca eradication efforts in Peru reduce economic activity and family incomes [9]. A study of the impact of India's trade liberalization on child labour in urban India found that children work more in cities and towns that had more employment in industries losing tariff protection [10].

The observation that children tend to work more during economic downturns, when the economic contribution of children is lower, may seem surprising. Even when the net economic contribution of the working child is small, it may be important to the welfare of a poor family. A family surviving on a dollar a day doubles its standard of living if a working child brings an additional dollar into the household. In fact, children often work more during a family crisis when the family's need for income is likely to be elevated relative to the family's norm. A study of rural families in Tanzania found that families turn to child labour to help deal with crisis on their farm [11], while another documents that children in northern Mali fill in for their mother when she is ill [12]. Children assume their mother's family responsibilities and replace her in the family farm and business.

The decision to work does not only depend on the potential economic contribution of the child. It also depends on the perceived returns to other available activities. Schooling is not the only alternative use of a child's time outside of work. Leisure and play are important components of how children spend their time and may be critically important for child development. In fact, the debates over child labour in the United States and Great Britain during the later part of the nineteenth century and the early part of the twentieth century emphasized the value of leisure and play as reasons why children should not work. A right to play is codified in Article 31 of the 1989 Convention on the Rights of the Child [13].

In the modern era, schooling is typically viewed as the most important alternative use of a child's time outside of work. This is not always a logical view as child labour is most prevalent in the poorest places where schools can be absent or lacking in teachers and educational materials. Overall, the child's potential economic contribution must be weighed against the return to education and how the family values that return. Schooling costs can play a critical role in this calculation. One recent study of rural India argues that the child's most important economic contribution may be the avoidance of schooling costs that result from attending school [14].

There is a conspicuous lack of direct evidence showing a connection between the additional income children can expect to earn in the future if they acquire more education and child labour. However, some of the apparently most effective interventions against child labour work by increasing the returns to education. Conditional cash transfer programmes give poor families cash for sending their children to school. Programmes like Mexico's *Progresa* have been shown to substantively alter child time allocation, increasing schooling and sometimes decreasing child labour at the same time [15]. By increasing returns to education and reducing poverty, conditional cash transfers appear to both reduce the net economic gain from having the child work and diminish the family's need for that economic contribution.

Health in the economics of child labour

Health-related issues enter into the discussion of the economics of child labour in three ways. First, adult illness may lower living standards, motivating poor families to send their children to work to compensate for some of the lost adult income. Second, adult illness may increase the return to children working inside their own family as families need the child to fill in for the lost worker or the adult illness creates new demand for the child's labour. Third, the possibility that the child becomes ill or injured during work can influence how the family values the child's potential net economic contribution from working.

There is a great deal of evidence from a wide variety of country contexts that poor families have difficulty buffering illness and injury shocks to adult earners. Families become poorer when an adult earner loses his ability to work. The evidence discussed in the previous section suggests a strong link between living standards and child labour. Hence, we expect adult illness and injury to lead to more child labour. The evidence from northern Mali that children fill in for their sick mother, mentioned above, supports this hypothesis [16]. A recent study of rag-pickers and porters in Nepal suggests that parental morbidity may be especially important for understanding entry into worst forms of child labour [17]. Porters are five times and rag-pickers four times more likely to have disabled parents than other wage working children in Nepal.

It is not obvious that parental morbidity will lead to more participation in worst forms of child labour in general. Family illness and injury may alter the return to work inside the household. Sometimes changes in the return to work might draw children into the labour market. At other times, another adult might fill in for the ill or injured in the formal labour market, causing the child's labour to be more valuable in household duties and chores. The family may also need the child to take care of the ill or injured. Hence, the effect of a decline in income associated with poor adult health or injury is likely to push the child towards working. With all of these different ways that adult morbidity might interact with child time allocation, we cannot draw generalizations about how children will be affected by adult morbidity.

Less ambiguous is the impact of the child's illness or injury potential on child labour. The threat of illness and injury makes the child worse off. The threat of illness or injury makes it less likely that the child will work in that task by lowering the welfare improvement associated with the child's potential economic contribution, provided these threats are observable and understood by whomever is making child labour decisions. These effects will be more readily observable with injuries but perhaps less so with chronic illnesses such as asthma.

Illness and injury threats reduce a person's willingness to take a job unless these threats are compensated. The existence of compensating wage differentials for unpleasant or risky tasks is documented in labour market data [18]. Adults in riskier occupations are paid more even though public health researchers often find that adult workers cannot accurately detail all of the risks they face. Evidence of compensating wage differentials does not appear to exist for working children. It is possible, in theory, that the same factors that lead adults to be paid more in risky occupations also influence the wages of children as children often work by their parent's side.

There are several salient issues with children that can lead them to be exposed to risks that are not compensated. We begin with two issues related to who has agency in the child labour decision. First, children rarely have complete agency over their work decisions and parents may not be perfectly altruistic. Parents may not understand the risks faced by their children and they may value the risks in the same way that a fully informed person would for him or herself. Second, children may have too much agency and do a poor job of appropriately assessing risks. The feeling of invincibility that often accompanies adolescence may cause children to undertake more risk than adults would be willing to bear, and it can be challenging for an adult to affect more appropriately cautious or safe behaviour.

Another issue that may lead to risks that are not fully compensated is that children and adults may neglect issues associated with child longevity. Children live longer than adults. Hence, any occupational risk associated with a job that may lead to permanent disability is more costly for a child than an adult. Moreover, children who start work earlier will be exposed to health and injury risks for longer. An adult decision-maker may not understand the long-term costs of their child's work.

If the present discounted cost of injury to a child is greater because of longevity, then children should receive a larger compensating wage differential than adults. This would appear as a larger premium for children in a task than for adults. That is, children should be expensive relative to adults in the risky activity. So long as there is a riskless activity, children should specialize in that. The fact that children participate in risky activities suggests that longevity issues are either not fully considered, not clearly understood, or both. As pointed to elsewhere in this book, it is difficult for those with significant expertise to understand the risks faced by young workers. Many serious hazards may have effects that go entirely unobserved or may not be attributed to their cause (i.e. work).

This later argument assumed that children are free to switch jobs like adults. Indeed, the whole idea of a compensating differential presumes that there are competitive labour markets for child labour. However, child labour may not fully compensate for health and safety risks, because children often do not participate in competitive labour markets. When working for a parent, children are often not free to leave if they are not appropriately compensated for the risks they face. Similarly, when a child works away from home, the employer often bears a responsibility for caring for the child that may lead to an analogous degree of immobility. When labour is effectively bonded, it has no leverage to affect a compensating differential for the risks faced.

Thus, there are many reasons to think that health and injury risks are not compensated in children despite the absence of concrete evidence on this point. We would expect these uncompensated risks to cause children to be less likely to work in tasks with risks of illness or injury. However, information can often be a problem. When children work away from their parent, the person who makes decisions about the terms of the child's employment may lack or disregard information about working conditions. Hence, risks are not compensated. When combined with the effectively bonded status of many child workers, it is possible that they may face risks that no adult would tolerate, that they go uncompensated for such risks, and that the person making decisions about whether the child should work was uninformed about these risks or powerless to alter the situation for themselves and/or their child.

Are working children less healthy as children or adults?

The previous section argued that caregiver ill health generally makes it more likely that the child works and can also influence how the child works.

Health and injury threats to the child worker that are known and understood should reduce the likelihood that the child works provided these risks are understood by concerned decision-makers.

Work-induced illness and injury may directly worsen the health status of child labourers. There are many reasons other than work-induced illness or injury to suspect worse health outcomes for child labourers. Working children typically face greater caloric demands than non-working children. When these are not met with increased nutrient intake (either because of the circumstances of the child's work, or the parent's lack of awareness about nutrition-related concerns), work may leave the child more vulnerable to illness, injury, and a lifetime of health issues. Working children may also suffer health consequences by foregoing the health and nutritional knowledge usually acquired in school. This may be uncompensated, because parents and children are unaware of the value of this information when they themselves have not received it. This is an example of another setting where the health-related costs of work are unknown to the person making child labour decisions.

The scope and limitations of studies on child health are discussed in other chapters. The question of the long-term consequences for adult health of working while young receives less attention elsewhere in this volume, and it is potentially of great importance for understanding the intergenerational transmission of poverty.

There are at least two basic classes of mechanisms through which a child's labour status may influence adult health. First, physical injury at work may lead to health problems that survive into adulthood. The injuries may be immediately evident to the child (e.g. a crushed foot) or may take years to become evident (e.g. exposure to toxins). Second, psychological stress or trauma at work in childhood may lead to health problems in adulthood.

Speculation about this second mechanism owes to the psychology literature which shows a strong correlation between stress in childhood and the persistence of mental disorders such as depression, anxiety and panic disorders, and schizophrenia, or even health problems such as diabetes, heart disease, and immune disorders [19]. There is a debate over the interpretation of this evidence as there is a strong correlation between severe stress in childhood and stressful life events in adulthood [20], but some argue that this association reflects that childhood traumas induce a vulnerability to the effects of stress later in life. Most of this research focuses on stresses like the loss of a parent and severe physical abuse at very young ages, so whether this evidence is relevant for typical child labour is an open question. For example, a recent study of the psychological impacts of forced abduction into the military among children from northern Uganda finds little evidence of sustained psychological distress after the end of conflict in child combatants relative to non-combatants [21].

Two recent studies consider whether child labour impacts future adult health. Individuals in Brazil who start work earlier have worse self-reported health statuses as adults [22]. The younger a person starts working, the greater the chance that the individual reports being ill as an adult. This finding may reflect something about the impact of child labour on child health and how that persists into adulthood, the impact of education on adult health, the impact of income on adult health, or something about the child's or adult's environment associated with both youthful work and adult health. A subsequent analysis of this data finds that the negative association between adult health and child labour disappears completely when one controls for education [23]. This might reflect that the lack of education is the underlying causal mechanism, or that early entry into the workforce and a lack of schooling are correlated jointly with entry into more hazardous occupations.

Public policy, health, and child labour

Public health enters the discussion of the economics of child labour because of the impact of caregiver health on the decision to work and because of the impact of work on child health and vice versa. On average, the impact of work on the health and injury status of working children has been difficult to identify in the data. There are many cases, discussed elsewhere in this volume, where work exposes children to health and safety risks, and there are several places in the preceding discussion where there may be a strong case for public intervention because of the health and safety risks of working.

Health and safety issues are more salient for working children than adults. The person making decisions about child labour (a parent, the family, the child, a third party) may not fully understand or take into account the impact of the work environment on the child's welfare. This could arise because of a lack of altruism, poor information about the work environment, difficulties in understanding the health effects of work, a lack of education, or myopia that does not properly weigh future consequences. Child labour's immobility leaves it especially susceptible to uncompensated health and safety risks.

The implications of these issues for economic policy are substantive. These agency and market power arguments can be used to make a case for government intervention against child labour where the government acts on behalf of the child. Externalities and information problems create a separate economic justification for government intervention even when the person making decisions about how the child spends her time has the child's best interests at heart. For example, a distinct argument for government intervention comes from the externalities created by an elevated incidence of illness and injury. Weak children with poor health or unhealthy work environments may contract and spread diseases that leave everyone worse off (e.g. tuberculosis, flu, HIV/AIDS). Injured children, who are unable to work or whose productivity is diminished, face a lifetime of depending on others for support. Both these costs are borne by the society and will not be internalized by the person making child labour decisions.

What economic policy tools are available if a case can be made to justify their use? Enforced prohibitions on certain types of work would reduce the incidence of illness and injury from the prohibited work category, but such labour regulations do little to address the factors that push children into that work to begin with.

A comprehensive approach to the problems of public health in child labour would consider both the health consequences of work and the role morbidity and mortality play in pushing children into work. This chapter has highlighted the important role that caregiver illness may play in motivating children to enter risky work in the first place. Efforts to strengthen social safety nets have considerable promise injury and illness in work. The recent growth of conditional cash transfer programmes in poor countries is one promising avenue for strengthening social safety nets in ways that both ameliorate poverty and create positive incentives for caregivers to invest in the human capital of their children.in keeping children out of work in general so that they are never exposed to risks of their children.

References

1 United Nations Children's Fund. Monitoring the situation of women and children. Available at: http://www.childinfo.org/mics3.html

2 Edmonds E, Pavcnik P (2005). Child labor in the global economy. *Journal of Economic Perspectives*, **19**:199–220.

3 Edmonds E (2008). Child labor. In Schultz TP, Strauss J (eds), *Handbook of Development Economics*, Vol. 4, pp. 3607–3710. Amsterdam: Elsevier Science.

4 Menon M, Pareli F, Rosati F (2005). Estimation of the contribution of child labour to the formation of rural incomes: An application to Nepal. Working Paper no. 10. Rome, Italy: Centre for Household Income, Labour and Demographic Economics.

5 Manacorda M, Rosati F (2008). Industrial structure and child labor: Evidence from Brazil. Working Paper no. 42. Rome, Italy: Understanding Children's Work.

6 Cockburn J, Dostie B (2007). Child work and schooling: The role of household asset profiles and poverty in rural Ethiopia. *Journal of African Economics*, **16**:519–563.

7 Basu K, Das S, Dutta B (2007). Child labor and household wealth: Theory and empirical evidence of an inverted-U. Working Paper no. 139. Cambridge, MA: Bureau for Research and Economic Analysis of Development.

8 Duryea S, Lam D, Levison D (2007). Effects of economic shocks on children's employment and schooling in Brazil. *Journal of Development Economics*, **84**:188–214.

9 Dammert A (2008). Child labor and schooling responses to changes in coca production in rural Peru. *Journal of Development Economics*, **86**:164–180.

10 Edmonds E, Pavcnik N, Topalova P (2009). Child labor and schooling in a globalizing world: some evidence from urban India. *Journal of European Economic Association*, **7**:498–507.

11 Beegle K, Dehejia R, Gatti R (2006). Child labor and agricultural shocks. *Journal of Development Economics*, **81**:80–96.

12 Dillon A (2008). Child labor and schooling responses to production and health shocks in northern Mali. Discussion Paper no. 755. Washington, DC: IFPRI, Development Strategy and Governance Division.

13 United Nations Children's Fund. Convention on the rights of the child. Available at http://www.unicef.org/crc/

14 Edmonds E, Pavcnik N, Topalova P (forthcoming). Trade adjustment and human capital investments: Evidence from Indian tariff reform. *American Economic Journals: Applied Economics*, forthcoming.

15 Fiszbein A, Schady N, Ferreira F, Grosh M, Kelleher N (2009). *Conditional cash transfers: Reducing present and future poverty*. Washington, DC: World Bank Publications.

16 Dillon A (2008). Ibid.

17 Edmonds E (2010). Selection into worst forms of child labor. *Research in Labor Economics*, **31**, forthcoming.

18 Rosen S (1986). The theory of equalizing differences. In Ashenfelter O, Card D (eds), *The Handbook of Labor Economics*, Vol. 1, pp. 641–92. Amsterdam: Elsevier Science.

19 Heim C, Nemeroff C (2001). The role of childhood trauma in the neurobiology of mood and anxiety disorders: Preclinical and clinical studies. *Biological Psychiatry*, **49**:1023–1039.

20 Horwitz W, Widom C, McLaughlin J, White H (2001). The impact of childhood abuse and neglect on adult mental health: A prospective study. *Journal of Health and Social Behavior*, **42**:184–201.

21 Blattman C (2006). The consequences of child soldiering. Working Paper no. 22. New York: Households in Conflict Network.

22 Kassouf A, McKee M, Mossialos E (2001). Early entrance to the job market and its effects on adult health. *Journal of Health Policy and Planning*, **16**:2–20.

23 Lee C, Orazem P (2010). Lifetime health consequences of child labor in Brazil. *Research in Labor Economics*, **31**, forthcoming.

Chapter 5

The child labour–education–health connection

David Post

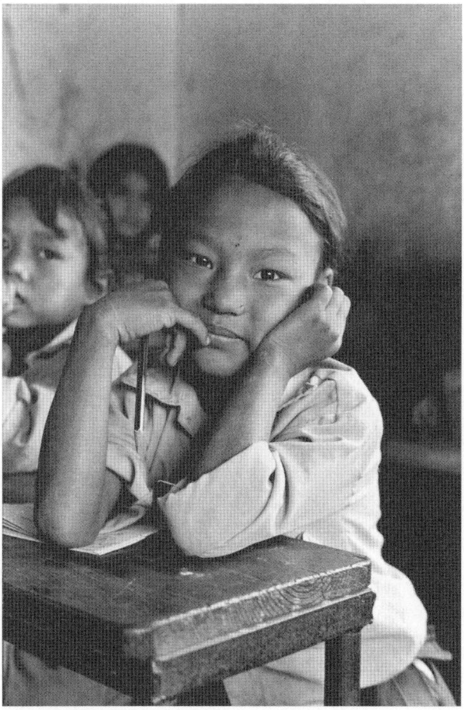

School children, Nepal

Introduction

Schools are often the main alternative to intensive child labour. Thus it is important, when considering child labour regulation from a public health perspective, to see the connections between the health of children and communities, on the one hand, and the availability of good schools and full-time participation in quality education on the other. Clearly, many types of work done by children ultimately harm their own health and that of their communities. Elsewhere in this volume, policy researchers and child advocates examine the *direct* consequences of work and the overall impact of child labour (net of any income or skills generated) for the physical integrity, nutrition, and survival of children and families. The emphasis of this chapter is on one of the most important *indirect* effects of child labour. Indirectly, children's work is harmful for health when such work precludes full-time education and thereby impedes mastery of the skills needed for healthy development. These consequences of work stem from the child's participation in or absence from quality schooling, assuming that such quality schooling would be accessible for them.

Following the worldwide ratification of the Convention on the Rights of the Child, access to schooling today is acknowledged as a universal right. But, in addition to rights-based arguments for education, there are powerful arguments against child labour based on the positive consequences of reducing children's work and increasing their learning because intensive work diminishes their likelihood of school successes. True, this association is not always a causal relation. Being in school does not invariably reduce the likelihood of working among children; and working full time does not always lessen the chances for school success.

Often the allocation of time and energy to schooling and working is simultaneously determined as families and children consider the current and future costs and benefits of different uses of the child's time. These decisions weigh the availability of quality and affordable education. Education can be very costly (in terms of books, uniforms, forgone earnings), even when the direct fees are low. The material benefits from education are not always obvious to families and – apart from school feeding programmes, discussed below – those benefits may come far in the future. One goal of public policy is to ensure that families make the kinds of choices they would want (and that the child would want) in the event that complete information about the full benefits and costs were available to all. In this sense, it is necessary to consider the individual and community health benefits to education because such benefits might be invisible to struggling families. If families and communities appreciated the full benefits of schooling, they would be less willing to permit children to work at an early age.

The political backdrop for considering the work–school–health connection is the strategic shift over the past decade by the International Labour Organization (ILO) and some countries as they deemphasized the ILO's Minimum Age Convention, 1973 (no. 138). Convention 138 included blanket prohibitions against nearly all forms of child labour during the age when school is compulsory. However, because Convention 138 was not ratified by many of the Southern nations where child labour is widespread, a new campaign and different strategy led to the adoption in 1999 of the Worst Forms of Child Labour Convention (no. 182). The mobilization and attention generated through the national campaigns to ratify Convention 182 have enabled proponents to secure also the ratification of Convention 138, but much of the emphasis today remains on the worst and most abusive forms of child labour.

What types of harm and how much harm are required before a type of child labour qualifies as one of the 'worst' forms of child labour and must be eradicated under Convention 182? Under the terms of Convention 138, work that impeded children's schooling was, by definition, illegal. ILO Recommendation 146 was to tie the age of legal employment to the age for the last year of compulsory education. Convention 182 is less clear on this point. It seems to sanction work that impedes children's education only if missing or failing school harms the child, and so the definition of a 'worst' form of child labour hinges on the empirical questions of how much educational harm there is from particular types and intensities of employment. Researchers have begun to examine the consequences to children's academic attainment as a result of their labour.

The remainder of this chapter first discusses the relationship between education and child labour, then, the evidence for a health-benefit from school participation. Next, it reviews the strategies used by governments and schools to attract and support working children in schools thereby, indirectly, reducing the incidence of child labour. Finally, a broader theoretical overview of the problem of school participation is presented, including non-governmental and grassroots organizing efforts on behalf of working children.

The education–child labour relationship

There may be situations in which some paid employment benefits academic achievement; the few comparative studies that have examined this relationship tend to find detrimental effects, even after controlling for the family resource effects known to increase both achievement and the likelihood of child labour [1, 2, 3, 4].

Studies of the individual and community health consequences of schooling specifically for working children are rare, although there is a voluminous literature on the general health benefit of education. Children's work, past a certain point in hours and intensity, can impede their academic achievement in schooling, and low academic achievement is likely to lead to reduced opportunities in the future. The types of work associated with negative learning outcomes, and the threshold points at which these effects ultimately appear, vary across and within nations. Less-healthy and academically weaker children are more likely to work, while they are less likely to attend school. Their self-selection makes the consequences of work unclear at times, and one study based on panel data from Vietnam found no increased likelihood of illness among children who had worked in past years [5]. When researchers take into account the endogeneity of school participation among students – the fact that it may be promoted by the same factors that promote health-negative consequences of child labour have been found for students both in terms of their individual health in Indonesia [6] and their academic achievement in Indonesia, the Philippines, and other countries [7].

Schools themselves are important in considerations of child labour and public health because lower-quality schools are more likely to push students to seek alternatives. When children are needed to supplement scarce family income, then low-quality schools provide no countervailing incentive for families to maintain their children in school [8]. In contrast, high-quality and close-by schools can reduce the likelihood that children will work exclusively or in addition to their time in school. As discussed below, free breakfasts and lunches not only promote children's health directly, but also help retain them in school and lessen the likelihood that they must work.

The two-way relationship between child labour and school quality is important in discussions of child labour as a public health problem because, ultimately, child-friendly and high-quality education will promote school attendance. This promotion will subsequently affect the health choices, risk behaviours, and nutritional decisions made by adults. Literate and better-educated individuals can evaluate more realistically such hazards as smoking, unprotected sexual behaviour, and unhealthy diet for themselves and their own children.

What about the community effects of education as an alternative to child labour? In the aggregate, a better-educated adult population is likely to embrace more progressive and less traditional views on childhood and to embrace the rights of their own children to education. The acceptance of global norms and the expectations for children can also work in a feed-back loop to improve educational quality. National and global campaigns to provide quality education for all children can press local governments to improve schools and, thereby, lower the incidence of harmful child labour. The Education For All movement has forced governments to report on the progress they make toward this goal, and the public global discussion may positively affect the willingness of governments to back rhetoric with resources. The mediating role of schooling in children's individual and community health thus goes beyond the curriculum and pedagogy on healthy behaviour. The presence or absence of quality schools affects the ways that families allocate their children's time, even as these choices simultaneously determine whether or not children will receive an education.

The education–health relationship

Education – or its absence – profoundly affects the health of children and their communities via several much-studied paths. First, a child's own education can improve his or her own health. It can also improve the health of their future children by affecting the number of births, their timing, and the resources available for the next generation. Successful schools affect children's health both directly, through their own education, and indirectly, through their parents' education [9, 10]. Education increases income and the quality of healthcare afforded by increased income. It also increases knowledge on health topics and knowledge about how to acquire answers to future questions. Finally, greater education tends to equalize gender equity within the household.

Infants whose parents are educated are more likely to receive neonatal care, less likely to experience the increased mortality associated with large families and closely aged siblings [11], and more likely to receive continued care and attention through their toddler years [12]. Girls who have been educated are more likely to seek out medical help as adults, to care for minor illnesses correctly, and to provide their families with proper nutrition. As a result, these families experience lower infant mortality, lower child mortality, and better child health measures such as stunting and illness [13, 14].

Nutrition, already mentioned as a primary concern for child health and survival, has been strongly linked to parents' education in health studies focused on developing countries [15]. In Latin America and the Caribbean, child nutrition problems include not only wasting and stunting, but also a growing number of overweight children. The percentage of children under the age of 5 who are overweight is 4.4%, 1.1% higher than the average for developing countries [16].

Women's education, or its lack, is closely related to infant and child mortality in many countries [17]. Educated mothers are more likely to seek medical care, to be better informed about their children's nutritional requirements, and to adopt improved sanitation practices. The result is that their infants and children have higher survival rates and tend to be healthier and better nourished [18]. An infant born to an educated woman is more likely to survive until adulthood. In general, an educated woman is 50% more likely to have her children immunized against childhood diseases [19, 20]. The effect of a mother's education on her child's health and nutrition is so significant that each extra year of maternal education reduces the rate of mortality for children under the age of 5 by between 5 and 10% [21].

Moreover, communities with a large percentage of educated families have a better environment and offer more health services for everyone, as compared with communities of uneducated adults. Because the children of educated parents are themselves more likely to be educated, they make better choices about nutrition and healthy lifestyles [22]. As the Millennium Development Goals state: 'The education of young people merits the highest priority in a world afflicted by HIV/AIDS, because education is the most effective – and the most cost-effective – means of preventing' HIV/AIDS [23]. This is even more necessary in poorer countries where large proportions of children work rather than attend school.

Educated women generally wait longer to become sexually active, which limits their exposure to sexually transmitted diseases such as AIDS and delays the start of child bearing. This further increases survival rates for both themselves and the infant [24, 25, 26, 27]. In summary, education conveys physical health benefits that go beyond children to include their later families and communities. Communities have better nutrition, lower rates of disease, and lower mortality when future members receive more education. In a large random sample of Dominican women in 2002, important relationships were discovered between the education received by girls and public health indicators as these girls became adults [28]. For example, half of the women without formal education were ignorant of any of the symptoms of sexually transmitted disease.

Investigations of education and demography have produced a worldwide consensus that the number of years that girls spend in schooling reduces the number of children they are likely to bear. Education provides tools for children eventually to seek and to understand information about contraception. It further increases the value of time by women to pursue economic activity [29, 30]. It is equally clear, from the 1995 data collected internationally by the Demographic and Health Surveys, that fertility rates are substantially lower amongst better-educated women. The Demographic and Health Surveys study found that education affects fertility through a number of channels, including the delay of marriage, increased likelihood of using contraception, and decrease in desired family size [31].

One study in India revealed that a 10% reduction in female illiteracy reduced the infant mortality rate by 12.5 per 1000 births, evidence of a strong association between female illiteracy and infant mortality rates [32]. Another study in Bolivia similarly found that maternal education was the most widely reported correlate of infant and child mortality. Education is associated with better knowledge of, and access to, health care. Furthermore, education fosters more positive attitudes towards modern health care, higher socioeconomic status, and greater female autonomy [33].

Research on women's education and fertility in Brazil found that more educated mothers opt for 'quality' of childhood rather than 'quantity' of children [34, 35]. As more children survive, families reduce the number of children they have; desired family sizes decline, a process helped by the ready availability of contraceptives [36]. Education, and specifically the education of girls, tends to improve maternal health by its effects at both the individual and societal level.

How schooling can reduce child labour

Many incentives have been used to induce school attendance in place of child labour. These include: cash payments; school feeding programmes; payment of direct costs; voucher systems of school finance; apprenticeship programmes to give students a salary along with their schooling; and incentives to school administrators. In addition to these material incentives, governments and NGOs can increase the subjective valuation of education relative to work by sending a message about what types of behaviour are normative for families and communities.

Stipends and cash payments

One example of a stipend programme to decrease child labour and increase school participation is found in Mexico's 1997 Program for Education, Health, and Nutrition (PROGRESA). PROGRESA (later 'Oportunidades') was noteworthy because it was designed to attend to the integral needs of children and families living in poverty. The programme focused specifically on families in the lowest 20% of the income distribution who live in Mexico's poorest communities, comprising some 24 million persons. It aimed to integrate existing welfare programmes of education, health, and nutrition.

In a significant departure from most other school incentive programmes, PROGRESA established a different scale of stipends for girls and boys after they complete primary schooling (up to the primary level equal monetary incentives are awarded for girls and boys). Following the examples of targeted programmes in Bangladesh and Guatemala, where the World Bank piloted a special subsidization of education for girls, PROGRESA specifically targets girls' access to schooling, since they are more likely than boys not to be in school. Most poor Mexican girls who are out of school do not work for income; rather, they are more likely to perform non-paid domestic chores [37].

PROGRESA increased the rates of school participation, especially among girls [38]. This lends support to the assumption that a differential stipend for girls can help increase their school participation relative to boys, and that poverty has a more detrimental impact for girls than for boys. PROGRESA significantly increased enrolment and reduced employment among both boys and girls, with boy's labour-force participation decreasing up to 25% with respect to their participation prior to the programme and domestic work decreasing for girls [39]. It remains to be seen whether the participation by girls and boys will lead to lasting reductions in rates of child labour or whether, in contrast, working children simply add schooling to their existing responsibilities and reduce their amount of leisure. Further research in Brazil, discussed as a case study in this book, suggests that programmes providing stipends for school attendance also lower the incidence of harmful child labour.

The Food for Education Programme was implemented in Bangladesh in 1994. Grains (wheat) were provided to poor rural families on a monthly basis, conditioned on children being enrolled in school. Families could freely trade the food received through the programme for other goods. Evaluating the impact of Food for Education on child labour and schooling, Ravallion and Wodon found a positive effect on school attendance and a negative effect on child labour [40]. However, the decrease in the amount of time spent in labour corresponded to a small share of the increase in schooling time, indicating that time dedicated to school is mainly subtracted from leisure and not from work time.

Economic non-market benefits for health

For many children in the world, education has direct costs to parents, above and beyond the opportunity costs of forgone earnings. There are many other children who would like to attend school but who cannot afford to pay for transportation, uniforms, necessary school supplies, or school lunches. Even when nations have pledged to make basic education free and compulsory for all, there are many hidden costs that prevent families from sending children to school. In simple economic terms, even when families are convinced that schools produce positive long-run returns to their investment (through payment of foregone earnings and direct costs), many families do not have the resources available to make this investment.

Free lunch and free breakfast programmes are one way to reduce the costs to families of sending children to school. In many countries, these interventions are justified in terms of nutritional supplements to poor diets. Benefits are measured in terms of children's growth and health. In addition to these clear benefits, there is also evidence that the poorest parents respond favourably to feeding programmes by sending children to school. In other words, there would be expected benefits to the poorest children in terms of increased school participation and reduced labour. In Kenya, according the ILO, the World Food Programmes (WFPs) provided lunch for 357,400 primary and pre-primary school children in 1362 schools. Because of the programme's success, WFP will expand the school lunches to 1,052,000 school age children.

In an assessment by the ILO, 'These WFP school lunch programs have proven instrumental in encouraging school attendance, limiting dropout rates, and maintaining the caloric intake for nutritionally vulnerable students' [41]. Easton and

Fass studied two poor communities in Haiti [42]. They discovered that the most basic diet, one that would include 1500 calories and 30 grams of protein for each adult in these communities, would cost the equivalent of US $4.80 per month, or about half of the average income among the participants of this study.

A critically important benefit for students in the neighbourhood of St. Martin was the average daily food ration of 800 calories and 40 grams of protein in school meals. For a household with the average number of three children in school, this would represent the equivalent of US $5.10 per month, over half of the average income of many families. In this context, according to Easton and Fass, 'a poor family would have been irrational not to send as many children to school as possible' [42]. This high consumption benefit of school attendance was sufficient to overcome the very high returns on out-of-school activities (high because the investments needed for them were minimal). Another benefit of school feeding programmes is that they lend legitimacy to education institutions and strengthen the faith of communities that schools are genuinely important alternatives to child labour.

Apart from the possible inefficiencies of this approach because feeding programmes are available to all rather than to the very needy, there are administrative risks to this approach. The control over the resources to feed millions of children, especially when channeled from donor agencies and government, becomes contested in a political control struggle. Corruption and waste can result without careful oversight.

Education reforms that combine the principles of demand and supply-driven incentives

School finance reform, though never undertaken specifically to assist children working in difficult circumstances, certainly has an impact on child labour and, consequently, on community health. Decentralization of school finance is one way that education ministries try to make localities accountable for ensuring that children attend school. In nations where all teachers and all school directors are employed by the central government, there is little opportunity for communities to participate and give feedback to schools that would improve the experience of education. There is very little incentive for schools to intervene and help out-of-school, working children in nations where school budgets are allocated in a centralized, politicized process, and where budgets do not depend on how many children actually go to school from day-to-day (or, in some countries, even from year-to-year).

Many educators assist working children who try to attend and succeed in school. But, recognizing that altruism is a feeble timber for the construction of strong programmes, the benefits of a school finance system that makes the enrolment of working children in the self-interest of the school rather than dependent on the care by individual teachers or administrators should be considered. In the United States, this has long been accomplished by a funding formula which counts the numbers of students in school every day and then distributes state money to school districts depending on the average daily attendance. For this reason, districts gain money for themselves when children who previously did not attend school are persuaded to do so.

In most countries where abusive child labour is a problem, the system for financing education is quite centralized. Given that most schools are grossly under-funded, over-crowded, and under-staffed, teachers face larger numbers of students than they can accommodate. There is very little reason to expect any but the most saintly teachers and school directors will want to attract additional students, or to worry about the dropout rates of students who decide to leave school. A 'triage' mentally pervades most schools in countries where significant numbers of children are exploited and abused at work. Teachers and school directors reconcile themselves to the idea that they can save only a fraction of the at-risk students who enter the system, and will not be able to help many others for whom there are simply insufficient resources. Research is needed to find whether children are at less risk of working in countries where their school attendance brings greater school funding.

Official curricula and NGO mobilization against abuse and exploitation of children

For poor and marginalized families and their children, schools represent the major contact point with the dominant culture and legal norms. The legitimacy that schools offer in their views about healthy activity for children carries symbolic as well as technical or informational meaning to families and students. Even when parents do not themselves receive lessons on child labour hazards, the parents' awareness of the importance of this issue is likely to increase simply when schools show concern about abusive labour.

The ILO's International Programme on the Elimination of Child Labour (IPEC) has undertaken a major project, 'Mobilizing Educators, Teachers, and Organizations to Combat Child Labour'. The project has been developed in Bangladesh, Brazil, Egypt, Kenya, the Philippines, Nepal, Paraguay, Peru, and Tanzania. The legacy of this effort is that teacher information kits are currently available from IPEC in English, Spanish, French, kiSwahili, and Arabic. They are currently being adapted for use in Brazil, Egypt, the Philippines, Paraguay, Peru, Tanzania, Indonesia, and Nepal.

In Nepal's Tribhuvan University, for example, the Faculty of Education has implemented curricula on social justice. Meanwhile, the Faculty of Social Work, at the St. Xavier campus, will include selected social justice issues into the curriculum of secondary schools in order to sensitize students on the issue of child labour, child rights, and gender equality. In Thailand, IPEC has supported a school intervention in 22 schools where there had been high drop-out rates. The active participation of teachers and of the community has been sought. Curriculum material about child labour was developed with local input so as to teach children about the health and safety impact of hazardous work, and about Thai labour laws and children's legal rights. According to IPEC officials, most of the children in the schools participating in this project finished their secondary school education, but no follow-up information is available yet to gauge the impact on their health.

Conclusions

The availability of child-friendly and high-quality education promotes school attendance and reduces participation in child labour. In addition to the direct benefits found by reducing intensive child labour, there are important indirect public health benefits for families and communities that are also evident from children's educational success. Few families think first or foremost about these health benefits. Parents are much more likely to consider whether or not schools are child-friendly, and whether or not graduates obtain good jobs, when they decide whether to forego their children's labour and permit full-time school attendance.

It follows that greater discussion about the health benefits of school success would incentivize families and children to dedicate their energy toward schooling and away from working. Where parents have discounted education as an alternative because schools are of poor quality, too unfriendly, or are not accessible, then a greater awareness of the health benefits of quality education could also cause families to exert political pressure to improve schools and promote access for all. As schools improved, so would community and child health, making more visible the connection between the two. This feedback loop could create a virtuous cycle, ultimately diminishing the reliance on child labour even without further legal regulation by local governments. To promote this virtuous cycle, leaders in the fields of education and public health would be advised to publicize the quality-of-life consequences of successful schooling: longevity, maternal and infant survival, and meaningful, safe, and productive work after the completion of education.

References

1 Heady C (2000). What is the effect of child labor on learning achievement? Evidence from Ghana. Innocenti Working Paper no. 79. Florence, UNICEF Innocenti Research Centre. Available at www.unicef-irc.org/publications/pdf/iwp79.pdf.

2 Knaul F (2001). The impact of child labor and school dropout on human capital: Gender differences in Mexico. In Katz EG, Correia MC (eds), *The Economics of Gender*

in Mexico: Work, Family, State and Market, pp. 46–84. Washington, DC: The World Bank.

3 Post D, Pong S (2000). Employment during middle school: the effects on academic achievement in the U.S. and abroad. *Educational Evaluation and Policy Analysis*, **22**:273–98.

4 Orezem P, Gunnarsson V, Sanchez M (2006). Child labor and school achievement in Latin America.*World Bank Economic Review*, **20**:31–54.

5 Beegle K, Dehejia R, Gatti R (2004). Why should we care about child labor? The education, labor market, and health consequences of child labor. Working Paper no. 10980. National Bureau of Economic Research.

6 Wolff F, Maliki (2008). Evidence of the impact of child labor on child health in Indonesia, 1993–2000. *Economics and Human Biology*, **6**:143–69.

7 Post D, Pong S (2009). Student labour and academic proficiency in international perspective. *International Labour Review*, **148**(1–2):93–122.

8 Boyden J, Ling B, Myers W (1998). What works for working children. Stockholm: UNICEF and Radda Barnen.

9 Macassa G, Ghilagaber G, Bernhardt E, Diderichsen F, Burström B (2003). Inequalities in child mortality in Mozambique: differentials by parental socio-economic position. *Social Science Medicine*, **57**(12):2255–64.

10 Gebre-Egziabher K, Hogan DP (2001) war, famine, and excess child mortality in Africa: The role of parental education. *International Journal of Epidemiology*, **30**:1–9.

11 Whitworth A, Stephenson R (2002). Birth spacing, sibling rivalry and child mortality. *Social Science Medicine*, **55**(12):2107–19.

12 Levine RA, LeVine, SE, Richman A, Tapia Uribe FM, Correa CS, Miller PM (1991). Women's schooling and child care in the demographic transition: a Mexican case study. *Population and Development Review*, **17**:459–96.

13 Behrman JR, Wolfe BL (1984). More evidence on nutrition demand: Income seems overrated and women's schooling underemphasized. *Journal of Development Economics*, **14**:105–28.

14 Mellington N, Cameron L (1999). Female education and child mortality in Indonesia. *Bulletin Indonesian Econonic Studies*, **35**(3):115–44.

15 Ayaya SO, Esamai FO, Rotich J, Olwambula AR (2004). Socio-economic factors predisposing under five-year-old children to severe protein energy malnutrition at the Moi Teaching and Referral Hospital, Eldoret, Kenya. *East Africa Medical Journal*, **81**(8):415–21.

16 de Onis M, Blössner M (2000). Prevalence and trends of overweight among preschool children in developing countries. *American Journal of Clinical Nutrition* **72**(4):1032–9.

17 Levine R (1987). Women's schooling, patterns of fertility, and child survival. *Educational Researcher*, **16**:21.

18 World Bank (2001). *World Development Report*. Washington, D.C.

19 Department for International Development (DFID) (2005). *Annual Report 2005*. London

20 Desai S, Alva S (1998). Maternal education and child health: Is there a strong causal relationship? *Demography*, **35**(1):71–81.

21 The United Nations Children's Fund (UNICEF) (2004). The State of the World's Children. Girls, education and development. New York, USA.

22 Mirowsky J, Ross CE (1998). Education, personal control, lifestyle and health: A human capital hypothesis. *Research on Aging*, **20**(4):415–49.

23 World Bank (2005). *Millennium Development Goals, 2005.* http://web.worldbank.org/WBSITE/EXTERNAL/COUNTRIES/ECAEXT/0,,contentMDK:21722062~menuPK:258606~pagePK:146736~piPK:146830~theSitePK:258599,00.html

24 Friedman HL (1994). Reproductive health in adolescence. *World Health Statistics Quarterly*, **47**(1):31–5.

25 Gubhaju B (1986). Health problems in Nepal: With special reference to infant and child health, *Asian Profile*, **14**:165–74.

26 Chauliac M, Raimbault AM (1992). Adolescent pregnancy [Abstract]. *Dev Sante*, **98**:23–5.

27 Mehra S, Agrawal D (2004). Adolescent health determinants for pregnancy and child health outcomes among the urban poor. *India Pediatrics* **41**:137–45.

28 Achécar MM, Ramírez N, Polanco JJ, Ochoa LH, Lerebours G, García B (2002). República Dominicana. Encuesta Demográfica y de Salud (ENDESA). Santo Domingo

29 Easterline R, Crimmins E (1985). *The fertility revolution*. Chicago: University of Chicago Press.

30 Cochrane S (1979). *Fertility and education: What do we really know?* Baltimore: Johns Hopkins University Press.

31 Martin TC (1995). Women's education and fertility: results from 26 demographic and health surveys. *Studies in Family Planning*, **26**:187–202.

32 Gokhale M, Rao S, Garole V (2002). Infant mortality in India: Use of maternal and child health services in relation to literacy status. *Journal of Health Population and Nutrition*, **20**(2):38–47.

33 Heaton T, Forste R (2003). Rural/urban differences in child growth and survival in Bolivia. *Rural Sociology*, **68**(3).

34 Lam D, Duryea S (1999). Effects of schooling on fertility, labor supply, and investments in children, with evidence from Brazil. *The Journal of Human Resources*, **34**(1):160–92.

35 Gupta N, Leite IC (1999). Adolescent fertility behavior: Trends and determinants in northeastern Brazil. *International Family Planning Perspectives*, **25**:123–30.

36 UNDP Human Development Report (2003). New York, USA.

37 Post D (2001). Can targeted assistance make a difference for girls? *Gender and Society*, **15**:468–89.

38 Schultz T (2004). School subsidies for the poor: Evaluating the Mexican PROGRESA poverty program. *Journal of Development Economics*, **74**:199–250.

39 Emmanuel Skoufias E, Parker S, Behrman J, Pessino C (2001). Conditional cash transfers and their impact on child work and schooling: Evidence from the PROGRESA program in Mexico. *Economía*, **2**:45–96.

40 Ravallion M, Wodon Q, (2000). Does child labour displace schooling? Evidence on behavioural responses to an enrollment subsidy. *Economic Journal*, **110**:C158–75.

41 Oyuga B (1997). A study of action against child labor in Kenya. Kenya: ILO/IPEC.

42 Easton P, Fass SM (1989). Monetary consumption benefits and the demand for primary schooling in Haiti. *Comparative Education Review*, **33**:176–93.

Chapter 6

Social values and child labour

Virginia Morrow and Jo Boyden

Introduction

Social values are defined as the norms, ideals, and aspirations shared by people in specific locations and cultures. With regard to child labour these are the beliefs about children's development and the associated norms concerning the roles, responsibilities, and activities appropriate for girls and boys at different ages. The term 'child labour' is itself value laden, and not one that is likely to be used by children, parents, or communities in most parts of the world [1, 2].

Although the evidence base is not extensive, the importance of social and cultural values in children's work is beginning to be recognized within the child labour literature. Economists Patrinos and Shafiq describe what they refer to as a 'positive stigma' regarding children working, whereby some forms of work are approved of and encouraged in communities, and households take pride in work in a household business or farm, especially when combined with schooling [3]. Drawing on a number of studies and commentaries, this chapter explores how social and cultural values related to child development, gender, marriage, religion, and ethnicity may affect children's labour in low-income countries.

Child development

Different cultures have different ideas about how children develop and learn, and about the contributions children make to their families and communities. These ideas shape children's transitions through childhood as much as the expectations and experiences of childhood work [4]. In some communities, work is regarded as an important mechanism of learning, and children's roles and responsibilities reflect views about both their evolving competencies and their learning needs.

Children under age 5 years or so may be encouraged to engage in 'play-work', so that they can learn basic life skills through the observation and mimicking of elders but without any expectation of real responsibility [5]. Transitions in children's work often herald broader changes in their social status.

For instance, in Bangladesh children who work and are thought to be able to fend for themselves are not referred to as children, whereas children of the same age who remain at school do not leave childhood until puberty or beyond [6]. At the same time, insofar as it supports the fulfilment of boys' and girls' duties towards their family, child work is often regarded as reinforcing intergenerational collaboration and enhancing young people's social skills.

While there are many beliefs about children's capacities and limitations in relation to work, there are some commonalities across cultures. For example, it is generally believed that the very young lack certain physical, social, and cognitive attributes which are important in the successful accomplishment of work, so that they are encouraged and indulged when they practice work skills, without penalty for mistakes.

Children's physical strength and agility, their knowledge of the world, and their capacity to plan and organize their time is often thought to increase at around the age of 6 to 8 years [7]. Belief in children's evolving competence for work during middle childhood tends to be reflected in the growing complexity and degree of specialization in the tasks they undertake. By around the age 12 years, their work may become more demanding and they may have the sole responsibility for some activities as well as being admonished for poor performance [8]. Puberty is commonly regarded as the threshold of adulthood. At this point, children may assume a work load similar to that undertaken by adults; girls generally transitioning into adult roles and adulthood sooner than boys. Expectations that the young make a full contribution to household maintenance during the early teen years as well as attend school can become difficult to meet, resulting in high rates of school drop-out in many communities.

Gender

Ideas about gender have a powerful influence on child labour. Girls are less likely to be involved in leisure activities and to attend school, but more likely to engage in unremunerated work in the domestic sphere, to begin work earlier, and to work longer hours than boys [9]. Child labour mirrors adults' labour patterns in many respects in relation to gender, and children's roles are likely to be shaped by local assumptions about what girls and boys can or should do. Caring for small children tends to be a female occupation worldwide, whereas mining (for example) tends to be done by boys. Compared to boys, girls are typically expected to have a wider range of work responsibilities, often combining domestic chores with paid work and sometimes schooling [7].

Across most of Africa it is boys, and not girls, who tend to herd livestock. This is because this kind of economic activity can generate a considerable amount of cash. Income-generation is more likely to be a male business and tending livestock takes children away from the household sphere, where girls are more likely to work [10].

Gender roles are not fixed and gender roles in one society may be reversed in another. They may also reflect the birth order, the sex composition of the sibling group, the household composition, and the health status of other family members [7]. Punch, in her study of children's work in rural Bolivia, found that children assumed the gender roles of the opposite sex when the sex composition of the sibling group did not match the requirements for household survival [11].

It is often assumed that gender bias and related discrimination results in girls experiencing greater work-place risk than boys, and that certain risks, such as sexual exploitation, are associated almost exclusively with girls. However, boys are also susceptible to mistreatment at work, sometimes in dangerous occupations. In addition, social taboos against disclosure of infringements against boys may be extremely strong, especially where those infringements transgress the boundaries of 'acceptable' sexual conduct. Stereotypical assumptions about gender have led to a research and policy focus on girls, with far less known about the hazards confronted by boys.

Early marriage

Early marriage of girls may be considered a form of child labour itself, in the sense that young brides are often married to older men and expected to work hard and for long hours in the marital home. This is frequently under the close supervision of a mother-in-law and without the protections that are normally thought to exist in the natal home [12]. There is, however, no systematic research on the effects of this practice with regard to child marriage as a form of child labour.

The age of marriage may itself be affected by child work outside the home. Heissler, in her research with young people in Bangladesh who migrated to towns for work, suggests that the effect of domestic service, which may be undertaken by very young children, or work in the garment industry which is normally undertaken by older children, is to delay marriage rather than encourage it [13]. Girls worked to raise money towards their dowries. However, when they tried to find grooms, having worked was often regarded as an unattractive feature in girls so working children's families sought to downplay it.

In a study of 3000 girls in rural Bangladesh, Mahmud and Amin concluded that whether girls worked or got married were two separate decisions [14]. Based upon an analysis of two surveys of over 2000 Bangladeshi females aged 13–21 years conducted in 2001 and 2003, Amin and Suran found that 40% of the respondents reported some productive work, of which half was combined with childcare of their own children [15]. Although few in number, these studies suggest that there is no simple relationship between early marriage and child labour.

Religion

The interface between religion and child labour is explored in social anthropological research. It is not suggested that specific religions deliberately promote child labour, but rather that different religions give rise to powerful ideas about the appropriate activities of children.

Christianity has played an important part in shaping ideas about childhood, and throughout Africa colonial governments used children in mining and commercial agriculture, sometimes separating children from their parents [1]. Ideas dating from the colonial period continue to shape how childhood and children's roles are defined in post-colonial African societies today.

Over 40% of the population across the Saharan desert belt are Muslim. Bass suggests that historical Islamic practices have reinforced the functionality of child labour [1]. Although child labour is not specifically discussed in the Quran, children's begging is regarded as a service in exchange for Quranic education in Senegal and Gambia, and to a lesser extent in bordering countries. Referred to as *talibes* in Senegal and *almudos* in Gambia, these child workers are male and range from 7 to 13 years old.

Parents may place male children for some years with a *marabout*, or Quranic teacher, in order to learn the teachings of Allah. The children divide their time between begging and studying the Quran. Bass explains that Muslims have the responsibility to engage in *zakat*, or almsgiving, one of the five pillars of Islam. Begging is believed to instil a sense of humility and discipline in the child. The veneer of Islam may therefore have legitimized begging by Muslim children and insulated it from criticism. This practice is, however, increasingly viewed as unjust [1, 16].

The way that norms of *purdah* have been interpreted and observed within Islam also affects children's work contributions. Schildkrout's study of Muslim Hausa households in northern Nigeria described children's work as an integral part of women's strategies for managing market work and earning an income, as *purdah* barred women from public participation and children acted as intermediaries [17]. Women cooked snacks within their homes for sale by children to the public. Children were integrated into market life and set up their own businesses, often selling to other children. Hausa culture resisted universal primary education, because increasing school enrolment deprived parents, in particular mothers, of the presence of their children.

Caste

In India, the Hindu caste system is an important structuring principle and influence on the roles undertaken by children. Shirol, in a 1989–1990 ethnographic study of child labour in a village in Karnataka, India, described the complex relationship between social organization and child labour linked to the caste system [18]. He suggested that children took up work as part of enculturation processes. The nature of this work varied from family to family depending upon the caste status and its traditional occupation. Higher caste children typically worked to inherit traditional occupations rather than for wages. Lower caste children worked mainly for wages with less emphasis on developing traditional occupations. Through their social 'untouchability', Dalit children in particular were prevented from entering numerous relatively benign occupations with good income potential, and tended to be relegated to roles such as refuse collection and cleaning latrines. These jobs are stigmatizing and pose serious health risks. The Government of India has introduced numerous policy initiatives to try to reduce the effects of caste upon children's life chances [19].

Ethnicity

Ethnicity is a further dimension of social organization that affects child labour, although research into child labour amongst indigenous communities is sparse, particularly in African countries. Indigenous values and practices may favour children's involvement in what are perceived to be the more benign forms of labour because of a cultural belief that work contributes to learning and social integration. Heckt found that indigenous Mayan households in Guatemala valued children's work not only for income generation, but 'as a worthwhile activity in its own right' [21].

At the same time, these traditional values pre-date schooling, and most indigenous societies have a division of labour that incorporates all those who are able to work, such that children and adults can be understood as interdependent, and children's work is encouraged [7]. Bando *et al.* explored the relationships between child labour, school attendance, and indigenous households in Mexico. They analysed data collected in 1997 and 1999 to explore the effects of a conditional cash transfer programme on indigenous children's school attendance [22]. They suggest that the prevalence of child labour is greater in indigenous areas than in non-indigenous areas, and that children's contribution to total family income is substantial [22]. This contribution increases with age, and a child's income forms a larger part of the total family income in indigenous areas compared to non-indigenous areas. There is an expectation that indigenous children will be employed and not be in school because of language problems, school access problems, and 'cultural' differences. These cultural differences are not expanded upon.

In general, socialization practices amongst indigenous communities may be such that children are encouraged to contribute, although the types of contributions children make will vary. For more affluent children, the expected contribution is to study in school so as to get a better job in the future. For poorer groups, the expectation is that children will contribute to household maintenance, attending school only when feasible economically.

Children's work is also likely to be more common in indigenous populations because indigenous peoples tend to be the poorest and most marginalized socially and economically. At the same time, indigenous groups are often found in traditional economic sectors and informal occupations with low levels of technology, where children have historically played an important role. Larsen suggests that there are a large number of indigenous children engaged in the worst forms of child labour in certain countries in South Asia, Southeast Asia, and Latin America [20]. Indigenous and tribal children reportedly make up a large part of child labourers in risk areas, such as debt-bondage in South Asia, migratory agricultural wage labour in Central America and Mexico, and prostitution in Southeast Asia. In Latin America, indigenous children are reportedly twice as likely to work as their non-indigenous peers. In other words, indigenous children are more likely to work in hazardous forms of labour because of the extremely disadvantageous terms and conditions under which these populations are incorporated into national economies.

The relationship between social values and other determinants of child labour

Most child labour takes place within family agriculture. According to Panelli *et al.*, a number of factors contribute to this [25]. Agriculture is a 'traditional' occupation often associated with simple technology and considered to be safe and appropriate for the young. In reality, however, as is discussed elsewhere in this book, agricultural work can be extremely hazardous due to long hours of work, heavy loads, and exposure to risks such as extreme temperatures and toxic chemicals.

While work has long been regarded as important for informal learning and skills development, across the globe education is increasingly recognized as a means of ensuring success in the workforce. In some communities, child work and schooling are viewed as complementary, not competing activities; the aim being for children to take part in both [7]. Thus today, the great majority of children who work also attend school.

The social and cultural values that shape the relationship between education and work are complex, and may be compounded by the poor quality of education which may positively encourage child work. In India, formal education may have the effect of maintaining differentiation among social classes and to sustain a traditional Hindu social order. It does so by differentiating between the upper and lower castes. The Indian middle classes distinguish between the children of the poor who must be taught to work and their own children who must be taught to learn; the acquisition of manual skills being distinct from the acquisition of cognitive skills [26, 27].

While social and cultural values are important in shaping child labour in many contexts, all societies are affected by global political and economic trends and global values [1, 23, 24, 28]. The introduction of legal standards has been an important component of international child labour policy. Part of the reason that international, national, and local legislation has failed or been poorly promoted and enforced may relate to social and cultural values.

In recent years the focus of international legislation has shifted from the eradication of child labour and the enforcement of a minimum age to the elimination of the worst forms of child labour. Local values and local perceptions about childhood are important in understanding the possibilities for, and obstacles to, social change that can be brought about by legislation. Jaiswal, in a study of child labour in India, suggests that the traditional value system which holds that children ought to learn to work and help the family means that legislation is largely ineffective [26]. The perception of hazards and risk are all to a degree socially and culturally defined and will shape the impact the permissible boundaries of child labour. Adults and children know that there are limits to acceptable work and may comment if they feel children are being made to do work that is inappropriate for their age or gender. Communities may also determine and sanction what is appropriate and inappropriate [28].

Norms about what is tolerated in terms of harmful effects of child labour differ between communities and societies and will depend on many factors. These range from an awareness and understanding of work-related health risks to children to an economic necessity pushing children to work in hazardous occupations.

Children and adults do not always share the same values or views about child labour or education. Woodhead, in a study of the views of over 300 working children aged 10–14 years in Bangladesh, Ethiopia, the Philippines, and Central America, found that work and family security were interdependent. Children valued school above work, however, one of the most striking findings was the extent to which the wellbeing of children appeared to derive from the social affirmation given to their labour [29].

The African Charter on the Rights and Welfare of the Child, created in 1989 by the Organization of African Unity as a response to the UN Convention on the Rights of the Child (CRC), reflects culturally specific 'African' ideas about children and childhood. It emphasizes both children's right to protection from exploitation as well as their duties and responsibilities to their families, elders, and the national community by placing their physical and intellectual abilities at its service. Thus, collective rights are emphasized [10].

Conclusions

An understanding of the social and cultural contexts in which children's work takes place is crucial in order to address hazardous child labour. This does not mean that hazardous labour is acceptable because it is socially or culturally sanctioned. Rather, it is important to understand and acknowledge the perceptions of adults and children about early work in order to effectively engage communities. Children's involvement in work, whether hazardous or not, may be understood as an important mechanism through which children are integrated into their communities, facilitating their transitions to adulthood, as well as the acquisition of skills and knowledge that ensure basic survival.

Programmes and policies need to take account of the different perceptions of childhood as these underpin the understanding of whether or not children work, and under what conditions. This depends in part on social and cultural considerations that are not necessarily related to economic factors and that are not a mere function of the total labour demand in the household [10].

Incorporating social and cultural values into international policy and legislation is not straightforward. Nevertheless, harmful and exploitative situations do arise and to be properly addressed they need to be accurately examined in the appropriate social and cultural context to ensure that any intervention does not worsen the situation for children [2].

An understanding of the societal values held by states, communities, parents, and children themselves in specific locations needs to be incorporated into attempts to modify or limit the negative effects of labour on children's health and wellbeing. Working against communities is not effective, and in some societies children may consider that they have a right to work [30].

Finally, there needs to be an understanding that social values in relation to child labour are not fixed, but are dynamic and subject to change. They are not simply a reflection of local cultural practices but are affected by powerful forces related to globalization, development, and underdevelopment.

References

1 Bass L (2004). *Child labor in Sub-Saharan Africa*. Boulder, Colorado: Lynne Reinner Publishers.

2 Bourdillon M (2006). Children and work: A review of current literature and debates. *Development and Change*, **37**(6):1201–26.

3 Patrinos H, Shafiq M (2008). A positive stigma for child labor? Human Development Network Education Team Policy Research Working Paper no. 4697, World Bank.

4 Vogler P, Morrow V, Woodhead M (2009). Conceptualising and measuring children's time use: A technical review for young lives. Available at Young Lives, Oxford, www.younglives.org.uk (accessed 15 June 2009).

5 Briggs J (1990). Playwork as a tool in the socialization of an Inuit child. *Arctic Medical Research*, **49**:34–8.

6 Blanchet T (1996). *Lost innocence, stolen childhoods.* Dhaka: The University Press Limited.

7 Boyden J, Levison D (2000). Children as economic and social actors in the development process. EGDI Working Paper, Stockholm, Sweden.

8 Mendoza I (1993). Trabajo infantil rural en el Perú: la agricultura de esparagos en la Costa Norte (en valle de Viru). Geneva: ILO, INTERDEP/CL/1993/2.

9 Reynolds P (1991). *Dance civet cat. Child labour in the Zambezi Valley.* Athens, Ohio: University of Ohio Press.

10 Keilland A, Tovo M (2006). *Children at work. Child labor practices in Africa.* Boulder, Colorado: Lynne Reinner.

11 Punch S (2001). Negotiating autonomy: Childhoods in rural Bolivia. In Alanen L, Mayall B (eds), *Conceptualizing Child-Adult Relations*, pp. 26–36. London: Routledge.

12 McIntyre P (2006). *Married adolescents. No place of safety.* Geneva: WHO.

13 Heissler K (2009). On being 'good' in Bangladesh: Child labour, migration and choice in Madhupur Upazila. DPhil Thesis, Department of International Development, University of Oxford, Oxford.

14 Mahmud S, Amin S (2006). Girls' schooling and marriage in rural Bangladesh. *Research in Sociology of Education*, **15**:71–99.

15 Amin S, Suran L (2008). Terms of marriage and time-use patterns of young wives: Evidence from rural Bangladesh. Working Paper no. 10, Population Council, New York.

16 Tovo M (2008). Measuring the worst forms: The case of begging children in Senegal. Abstract of Paper presented at UCW Seminar, Madrid, September 2009.

17 Schildkrout E (2002). Age and gender in Hausa society: Socio-economic roles of children in urban Kano. *Childhood: A Journal of Global Child Research*, **9**(3):344–68. [Originally published in 'Sex and age as principles of social differentiation', ASA Monograph 17, ed. Jean La Fontaine, London, Academic Press, 1978.]

18 Shirol S (2000). *Child labour: A rural reality.* New Delhi: Classical Publishing Company.

19 Department of Education, Government of India (2006). *Sarva shiksha abhiyan: Fourth joint review mission.* New Delhi: Aide Memoire.

20 Larsen P (2003). Indigenous and tribal children: Assessing child labour and education challenges. Child Labour and Education Working Paper, ILO/IPEC, Geneva.

21 Heckt M (1999). Mayan education in Guatemala: A pedagogical model and its political context. *International Review of Education*, **45**(3/4):321–337.

22 Bando R, Lopez-Calva L, Patrinos H (2005). Child labor, school attendance, and indigenous households: Evidence from Mexico. Policy Research Working Paper no. 3487, World Bank.

23 Katz C (2004). *Growing up global. Economic restructuring and children's everyday lives.* Minneapolis: University of Minnesota Press.

24 Abebe T (2007). Changing livelihoods, changing childhoods: Patterns of children's work in rural Southern Ethiopia. *Children's Geographies*, **5**:77–93.

25 Panelli R, Punch S, Robson E (eds) (2007). *Global perspectives on rural childhood and youth: Young rural lives.* London and New York: Routledge.

26 Jasiwal P (2000). *Child labour: A sociological study.* Delhi: Shirpa Publications.

27 Kabeer N (2003). Depravation, discrimination and delivery: Competing explanations for child labour and educational failure in South Asia. In Kabeer N, Nambissan GB, Subrahmanian R (eds), *Child Labour and the Right to Education in South Asia: Needs versus Rights*, pp. 351–393. New Delhi: Sage.

28 Nesi G, Nogler L, Pertile M (2008). *Child labour in a globalised world. A legal analysis of ILO action.* Aldershot: Ashgate.

29 Woodhead M (2001). The value of work and school: A study of children's perspectives. In Lieten C, White B (eds), *Child Labour. Policy Options.* Amsterdam: Aksant.

30 Liebel M (2004). *A will of their own. Cross-cultural perspectives on working children.* London: Zed Books.

Chapter 7

International law and child labour

David Weissbrodt and Natalie W. Kohner

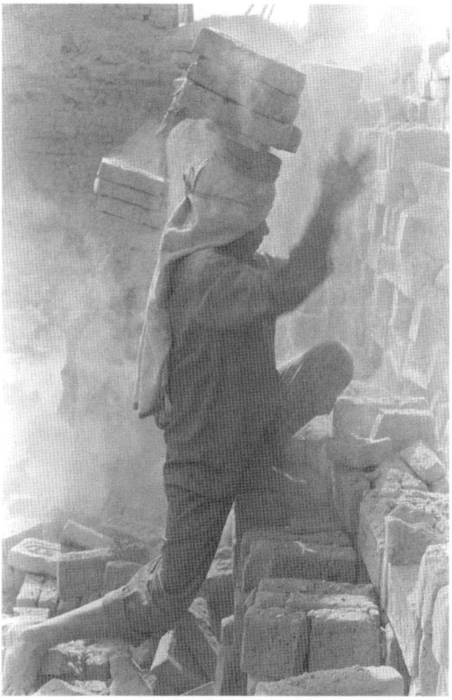

Brick worker, Nepal

Introduction

Legislation has been at the forefront of addressing child labour since the 19th century when public health campaigners in Europe and America first raised the moral and health issues that emerge from children working. The International Labour Organization (ILO), created in 1919 as part of the Treaty of Versailles that ended World War I, was established in part to ensure 'the protection of children and young persons' [1].

This chapter discusses the international legislation enacted with the purpose of regulating and modifying children's work and considers the impact of this legislation including how States are held to account. International child labour legislation focuses on children's rights as much as it does practical measures to regulate child labour. National legislation is not considered but is discussed in this book in the context of country-wide case studies. The development of hazardous child labour lists is also discussed elsewhere in this book. This chapter does consider the relationship between legislation and the other component parts of the public health model of child labour discussed throughout this book. In the case of legislation, this relationship is particularly evident with regard to human rights.

United Nations treaties concerning child labour

The United Nations Charter calls for the universal respect for human rights. The Universal Declaration of Human Rights was adopted by the United Nations General Assembly to authoritatively interpret the human rights obligations of the Charter and provides for special care and assistance for children [2]. Children's rights have been further delineated in multilateral treaties such as the International Covenant on Civil and Political Rights [3]; the International Covenant on Economic, Social and Cultural Rights [4]; and the Convention on the Rights of the Child [5].

Other United Nations treaties[1] contain provisions dealing with the rights of children. These are listed in Table 7.1. The Supplementary Convention to the Slavery Convention [6]. The ILO has also promulgated several treaties limiting child labour. In 1989, the United Nations adopted the Convention on the Rights of the Child, with several provisions combating child labour.

Article 24 of the International Covenant on Civil and Political Rights translates the general human rights obligations of the United Nations Charter into more specific treaty language and provides that; 'Every child shall have, without any discrimination as to race, colour, sex, language, religion, national or social origin, property or birth, the right to such measures of protection as are required by his status as a minor, on the part of his family, society and the State' [3]. This provision, which at the time of writing has been ratified by 164 nations, establishes a foundation for special protection for children due to their status as minors against abuse by the State, family, or society. Special protection is

1 A treaty is an agreement between two or more sovereign nations that has binding force. A convention is a treaty adopted by more than two nations – usually by many nations in the context of an international organization.

Table 7.1 United Nations Instruments

United Nations Instrument	Entry into Force
Universal Declaration of Human Rights	10 December 1948
Convention for the Suppression of the Traffic in Persons and of the Exploitation of the Prostitution of Others	25 July 1951
Supplementary Convention to the Slavery Convention	30 April 1957
International Covenant on Economic, Social and Cultural Rights	3 January 1976
International Covenant on Civil and Political Rights	23 March 1976
Convention on the Rights of the Child	2 September 1990
Optional Protocol to the Convention on the Rights of the Child on the Sale of Children, Child Prostitution and Child Pornography	18 January 2002
Optional Protocol to the Convention on the Rights of the Child on the Involvement of Children in Armed Conflicts	12 February 2002

further elucidated in Article 10 of the International Covenant on Economic, Social and Cultural Rights which affirms that:

> Children and young persons should be protected from economic and social exploitation. Their employment in work harmful to their morals or health or dangerous to life or likely to hamper their normal development should be punishable by law. States should also set age limits below which the paid employment of child labour should be prohibited and punishable by law [4].

That provision, ratified at the time or writing by 160 nations, recognizes that some working children are exploited or are required to do work that is life-threatening. Article 32 of the Convention on the Rights of the Child, ratified at the time of writing by 193 States parties, requires States to take action to prevent the worst forms of that labour:

1. States Parties recognize the right of the child to be protected from economic exploitation and from performing any work that is likely to be hazardous or to interfere with the child's education, or to be harmful to the child's health or physical, mental, spiritual, moral or social development.
2. States Parties shall in particular: (a) Provide for a minimum age or minimum ages for admission to employment; (b) Provide for appropriate regulation of the hours and conditions of employment; (c) Provide for appropriate penalties or other sanctions to ensure the effective enforcement of the present article [5].

Other United Nations treaties and other instruments apply to slavery and other forms of exploitation. The Universal Declaration of Human Rights condemns all forms of slavery in Article 4: 'No one shall be held in slavery or servitude; slavery and the slave trade shall be prohibited in all their forms' [6]. This and other fundamental provisions of the Universal Declaration constitute an authoritative interpretation of the United Nations Charter and customary international law. The Supplementary Convention to the Slavery Convention, with 83 States parties prohibits practices equivalent to slavery and defines those practices [7]. Article 1 of the Supplementary Convention applies to child labour and requests that states abolish and prohibit practices equivalent to slavery. Article 1(a) defines debt bondage as a form of labour equivalent to slavery.

Other United Nations conventions condemn the exploitation children face in the sex industry. The Convention for the Suppression of the Traffic in Persons and of the Exploitation of the Prostitution of Others with 93 States parties recognizes that children are often trafficked for prostitution [8]. The Optional Protocol to the Convention on the Rights of the Child on the Sale of Children, Child Prostitution and Child Pornography with to date 126 States parties recognizes child prostitution as one of the worst forms of child labour. Article 1 of that Optional Protocol calls for member States to prohibit child prostitution and Article 10 recognizes the need for member State cooperation on issues of child trafficking for sex [9].

In addition, recognizing that the recruitment of children into armed forces is one of the most insidious forms of child labour, Article 1 of the Optional Protocol to the Convention on the Rights of the Child on the involvement of children in armed conflicts provides that:

> States Parties shall take all feasible measures to ensure that members of their armed forces who have not attained the age of 18 years do not take a direct part in hostilities [10].

Article 2 of that Optional Protocol governs recruitment of children into the armed forces:

> States Parties shall ensure that persons who have not attained the age of 18 years are not compulsorily recruited into their armed forces.

International Labour Organization conventions concerning child labour

During its early history, and reflecting its founding principles, the ILO issued several conventions controlling the minimum age of workers. The earlier conventions concerned a minimum age for admission in specific occupations, then in 1976 Convention 138 proposed a general Minimum Age for Admission to Employment irrespective of occupation. This convention, however, met with some resistance and was not ratified by many countries. By 1998, when Convention 182 was being prepared, just 68 countries had ratified Convention 138.

In an effort to achieve greater consensus, in 1999, the ILO issued Convention 182 concerning the Prohibition and Immediate Action for the Elimination of the Worst Forms of Child Labour [11]. In contrast to Convention 138, Convention 182 was met with general consensus particularly with regard to child slavery, child prostitution, and child work in illicit activities as unconditional worst forms of child labour. This convention also defined hazardous child labour as a worst form of child labour giving particular attention to younger children. The convention, however, did allow for the types of work considered as hazardous child labour to be defined by national law. Interestingly, following the ratification of Convention 182 there followed a second wave of ratification of Convention 138 as many more countries defined a minimum age for admission to employment.

Article 3 of Convention 182 defines the worst forms of child labour:

(a) All forms of slavery or practices similar to slavery, such as the sale and trafficking of children, debt bondage and serfdom and forced or compulsory labour, including forced or compulsory recruitment of children for use in armed conflict;

(b) The use, procuring or offering of a child for prostitution, for the production of pornography or for pornographic performances;

(c) The use, procuring or offering of a child for illicit activities, in particular for the production and trafficking of drugs as defined in the relevant international treaties;

(d) Work which, by its nature or the circumstances in which it is carried out, is likely to harm the health, safety or morals of children. [11]

A total of 169 ILO member States have ratified Convention 182 and by consequence have a duty to take immediate action to prevent and end these forms of labour. Article 4 of Convention 182 allows States to determine, in consultation with employers and workers, and considering international standards, the forms of labour that are likely to harm the health, safety, or morals of children.

ILO Recommendation (no. 190) accompanying Convention 182 provides further guidance in Article 3(d) for determining which forms of child labour are likely to harm the health, safety, or morals of children [12]. Hazardous work is defined as:

(a) Work which exposes children to physical, psychological or sexual abuse;

(b) Work underground, under water, at dangerous heights or in confined spaces;

(c) Work with dangerous machinery, equipment and tools, or which involves the manual handling or transport of heavy loads;

(d) Work in an unhealthy environment which may, for example, expose children to hazardous substances, agents or processes, or to temperatures, noise levels, or vibrations damaging to their health;

(e) Work under particularly difficult conditions such as work for long hours or during the night or work where the child is unreasonably confined to the premises of the employer.

Moreover, Section 9 of the accompanying Recommendation no. 190 requires States parties to develop national mechanisms to monitor the prohibition and elimination of the worst forms of child labour. Section 11 requires States to cooperate with international efforts to prevent the worst forms of child labour and Section 12 requires States to criminalize conditions identified in Articles 3a, 3b, and 3c of Convention 182.

Article 7 of Convention 182 includes a special requirement on member States to both protect and rehabilitate children involved in the worst forms of child labour requiring that:

> Each Member shall, taking into account the importance of education in eliminating child labour, take effective and time-bound measures to:
>
> (a) Prevent the engagement of children in the worst forms of child labour;
>
> (b) Provide the necessary and appropriate direct assistance for the removal of children from the worst forms of child labour and for their rehabilitation and social integration;
>
> (c) Ensure access to free basic education, and, wherever possible and appropriate, vocational training, for all children removed from the worst forms of child labour;
>
> (d) Identify and reach out to children at special risk; and
>
> (e) Take account of the special situation of girls.

Other ILO conventions are applicable to child labour because they concern types of labour in which children are often involved. For example, Article 1 of the Convention concerning Forced or Compulsory Labour (ILO 29) requires each ratifying Member to suppress and not to make use of any form of forced or compulsory labour:

> (a) As a means of political coercion or education or as a punishment for holding or expressing political views or views ideologically opposed to the established political, social or economic system;
>
> (b) As a method of mobilising and using labour for purposes of economic development;
>
> (c) As a means of labour discipline
>
> (d) As a punishment for having participated in strikes; and
>
> (e) As a means of racial, social, national or religious discrimination. [13]

Article 5 of the Convention concerning the Protection of Wages (ILO 95) is also applicable to child labour since it requires that:

> Wages shall be paid directly to the worker concerned except as may be otherwise provided by national laws or regulations, collective agreement or arbitration award or where the worker concerned has agreed to the contrary. [14]

A full list of the ILO conventions that address child labour is given in Table 7.2. Ratification rates vary over time and an up-to-date table of ratification can be found at http://www.ilo.org/ilolex.

Implementation procedures

Treaties provide the formal legal means by which States may be held to some sort of international account. Just as important as ratification, however, are the actions taken by individual States with regard to implementation and enforcement of such legislation. As might be anticipated, States vary with regard to their duties of implementation and enforcement and sanctions are often quite weak. In addition, the application of treaties may be limited by declarations and reservations interposed by ratifying States. For example, in its declaration upon ratification, the Federal Republic of Germany declared that, domestically, the Convention on the Rights of the Child did not apply directly. The United States declared upon ratification that the International Covenant on Civil and Political Rights was not self-executing and that it therefore did not create a private right of action and could not be enforced in United States courts. While this declaration has been challenged, no United States court has found that treaty to be self-executing, or created legal remedies for its violation.

A number of measures are in place to encourage States to comply with their ratification duties regarding child labour. The following section illustrates some of the measures that have been taken to oblige or assist States in enforcement of child labour treaties.

A. Monitoring Committees: the Committee on the Rights of the Child; the Human Rights Committee; and the Committee on Economic, Social and Cultural Rights

The Convention on the Rights of the Child created a Committee, comprising 18 elected human rights experts to implement the provisions of the convention. Following Article 44 States parties must submit to the Committee reports detailing the measures they have taken to implement the convention within 2 years of ratification and then every 5 years afterwards. The Committee can also request additional information to supplement their reports. Following a

Table 7.2 International Labour Organization Instruments

ILO Convention or Recommendation	Entry into Force
Convention concerning Forced or Compulsory Labour (ILO no. 29)	1 May 1932
Convention concerning the Protection of Wages (ILO no. 95)	24 September 1952
Convention (no. 182) Concerning Worst Forms of Child Labour	17 June 1999
Recommendation (no. 190) Concerning Worst Forms of Child Labour Convention	17 June 1999
Convention (no. 5) Fixing the Minimum Age for Admission of Children to Industrial Employment	13 June 1921
Convention (no. 10) concerning the Age for Admission of Children to Employment in Agriculture	31 August 1923
Convention (no. 15) Fixing the Minimum Age for the Admission of Young Persons to Employment as Trimmers or Stokers	20 November 1922
Convention (no. 33) concerning the Age for Admission of Children to Non-Industrial Employment	06 June 1932
Convention (no. 58) Fixing the Minimum Age for the Admission of Children to Employment at Sea	11 April 1939
Convention (no. 59) Fixing the Minimum Age for Admission of Children to Industrial Employment	21 February 1941
Convention (no. 60) concerning the Age for Admission of Children to Non-Industrial Employment	29 December 1950
Convention (no. 79) concerning the Restriction of Night Work of Children and Young Persons in Non-Industrial Occupations	29 December 1950
Convention (no. 90) concerning the Night Work of Young Persons Employed in Industry	12 June 1951
Convention (no. 112) concerning the Minimum Age for Admission to Employment as Fishermen	07 November 1961
Convention (no. 123) concerning the Minimum Age for Admission to Employment Underground in Mines	10 November 1967
Convention (no. 124) concerning Medical Examination of Young Persons for Fitness for Employment Underground in Mines	13 December 1967
Convention (no. 138) concerning Minimum Age for Admission to Employment	19 June 1976

State report, Article 45 empowers the Committee to request aid for the country from the United Nations Children's Fund and other specialized agencies to assist the State in regard to any difficulties with implementation. Article 43 further empowers the Committee to make suggestions and recommendations for transmission to any State party concerned and reporting to the General Assembly, together with comments, if any, from States parties.

The Human Rights Committee and the Committee on Economic, Social and Cultural Rights have analogous procedures for receiving reports and producing concluding comments as to relevant provisions of their respective conventions including provisions concerning children's rights.

In its concluding comments on Greece, the Committee on the Rights of the Child noted the reports it received of street children being victims of sexual trafficking and abuse. The Committee also focused on Roma children. It reported that approximately 20% of children in Greece lived below the poverty line, with rates significantly higher for Roma children. Roma children, in particular, often lived in homes with no running water and with inadequate sanitation systems. The report was made publicly available and formally presented to the Greek Secretary-General of Welfare of the Ministry of Health and Welfare, who was also the head of the Greek delegation to the Committee. The recommendations the Committee, however, necessarily provided for Greece to interpret what its own national legal obligations were under the Convention on the Rights of the Child.

B. The Human Rights Council Special Rapporteurs

The UN Commission on Human Rights initially mandated in Resolution 1990/68 the creation of a Special Rapporteur to investigate the international exploitation of children and to make reports on the status of children and recommendations [15]. There are now several relevant thematic procedures with Special Rapporteurs on: the sale of children, child prostitution, and child pornography; trafficking in persons, especially in women and children; and contemporary forms of slavery. The Special Rapporteur on contemporary forms of slavery has identified the following practices within its mandate: debt bondage, serfdom, forced labour, child labour, child servitude, trafficking of persons and human organs, sexual slavery, children in armed conflict, sale of children, forced marriage and the sale of wives, migrant work, the exploitation of prostitution, and certain practices under *apartheid* and colonial regimes.

While each Special Rapporteur investigates and reports on a distinct subject matter, they follow similar reporting and implementation procedures. Special Rapporteurs can receive and investigate individual complaints. If they deem a complaint to be valid and identify imminent human rights abuses, they can issue an urgent appeal to a government. These communications and the government's response are reported annually to the Human Rights Council. Special Rapporteurs may also engage in country visits based on their thematic mandate and on information received about that country. Following the visit the Special Rapporteur issues a report and may make recommendations for improving human rights in their respective subject area.

For example, in 2007 a Special Rapporteur visited Mexico at the invitation of the government to investigate human trafficking. The Special Rapporteur met with government authorities, representatives of the judiciary, parliamentarians, representatives of non-governmental organizations, United Nations officials, and individuals. In Mexico City, the Special Rapporteur estimated that there were more than 25,000 children who were victims of child prostitution and in Guadalajara, he estimated that around 80 boys were child prostitutes. In Tijuana, he was unable to determine the number of children involved in child pornography or prostitution, but concluded that there were likely to be many as a result of demand from US residents either visiting Mexico or trafficking children into the United States. In Juárez, the Special Rapporteur documented over 200 murders of child prostitutes following physical and sexual abuse in brothels.

After the visit the Special Rapporteur issued a report documenting human trafficking and recommending policy and legal changes to discourage continued trafficking in women and children. In that report, he outlined the legal framework of rights protecting children in Mexico, the programmes in place to deter trafficking or to help already trafficked children, and the prevalence of child trafficking in various cities throughout Mexico. Finally, the Special Rapporteur suggested new approaches to combating child trafficking with specific regard to the programmes and policies already in place in Mexico.

While the Special Rapporteur commended Mexico on its openness to international scrutiny and its desire to combat child trafficking, he found that the programmes implemented by the country were too centralized. This approach hampered local enforcement in areas of the country cut off from the national government. The Special Rapporteur encouraged new non-governmental organizations to create programmes focused on child sexual exploitation that could better reach rural and tourist areas of the country. The Special Rapporteur also pointed out that the laws in place were commendable, but often not enforced due to police corruption and negligence. He recommended that child sex trafficking be addressed as part of the nation's organized crime problem. He further recommended that the all States make child sex prostitution a more serious crime along with better training and monitoring of police forces.

The Special Rapporteur therefore has a unique role in investigating and bringing human rights abuses with regard to child labour into the public domain. While the Special Rapporteur can, however, investigate, make recommendations, and publicize human rights abuses, he cannot compel changes in national policy.

C. International Labour Organization Monitoring and Investigations

The Constitution of the ILO provides for implementation of ILO conventions through several monitoring procedures. ILO Constitution Article 19 requires ratifying Member States to bring a convention before the relevant State authorities for enactment of legislation or other action within one year, or if there are exceptional circumstances, no later than 18 months from the closing of the session of the Conference. Article 19 also requires that ratifying States bring a Recommendation before the said competent authority or authorities, but requires 'no further obligation' on the Member State [16].

Article 22 of the ILO Constitution requires ratifying States to make a yearly report to the International Labour Office on the measures taken to implement the provisions of the convention. Article 25 allows the Governing Body of the ILO to determine that a report from a Member State is unsatisfactory and to publish that report and their response to it. Article 26 allows either Member States or the Governing Body of the ILO to issue complaints alleging that a Member State is not adequately implementing the convention. Once that complaint occurs, the Governing Body may communicate with the government in question or may appoint a Commission of Inquiry.

As outlined in Article when the Commission of Inquiry has fully considered the complaint, it must prepare a report with recommendations as to the steps required to address the complaint and the time-frame within which they should be taken. Following that report, Article 29 directs the Director-General of the International Labour Office to provide the report to any of the Member States concerned in the complaint and to publish the report.

D. International Labour Organization International Programme on the Elimination of Child Labour (IPEC)

In addition to its ratification, State reporting, and inquiry procedures based on provisions of the ILO Constitution, in 1992 the ILO adopted a more facilitative approach. It established the International Programme on the Elimination of Child Labour (IPEC) with the objective of progressively eliminating child labour through international assistance principally to governmental projects.

During 2006–2007 IPEC conducted 173 actions against child labour, some worldwide, and others specific to a certain region. IPEC programmes and projects help child labourers and children at risk of child labour, for example, by promoting primary education and helping families out of poverty. IPEC principally works to eradicate the worst forms of child labour by cooperating with governments and by making recommendations that do not have the force of law.

In addition, IPEC prepares resources and guides for policy- and law-makers to craft legislation and establish programmes for preventing and combating child labour. For example, in November 2008 IPEC produced a resource kit for policy-makers concerning the trafficking of children for labour exploitation. The resource kit contains five books with practical information on understanding human trafficking, designing policy responses, creating legal and political frameworks, taking remedial actions, and including examples of successful initiatives. In the legal and political frameworks book, IPEC focuses on the various roles of state organizations, non-governmental organizations, the media, civil society, and international organizations. So by providing a concrete resource on child trafficking, IPEC offers States that are serious about combating trafficking a practical starting point.

At the time of writing there is no published formal independent assessment of the impact of IPEC, but the establishment of IPEC is recognition that practical programmes and support measures addressing the wider determinants of child labour are just as, if not more important to combating child labour, than is formal State adherence to conventions and recommendations.

Conclusions

The scope of international legislation addressing child labour is wide ranging and in recent years the focus has moved from prohibition and minimum age requirements to the elimination of the worst forms of child labour and the identification of hazardous child labour. This statement is tempered with a proviso that age is in fact considered a key feature in the identification of hazardous child work. So age has come to be accepted as an important consideration, although individual countries may identify specific key ages.

Assessing the impact of international legislation is difficult. A mere head count of States parties to conventions says little about local enforcement and some States openly ratify treaties with statements limiting their applicability within those countries. This problem has now been recognized with the establishment of various bodies to supervise and encourage State enforcement.

Legislation in itself, as a means of securing child rights and tackling the worst forms of child labour is far from sufficient on its own. In recognition of the difficulties in using legislation and its enforcement to address child labour, the ILO has established the IPEC. IPEC comprises a wide programme of activities and measures. The aim is to work together with States and non-governmental institutions to address child labour within countries through tackling wider determinants such as poverty. Such an approach bodes well but remains to be formally assessed.

References

1 Treaty of Versailles, June 28, 1919, 225 Consol. T.S. 188, 2 Bevans 43.
2 Charter of the United Nations, June 26, 1945, 59 Stat. 1031, T.S. 993, 3 Bevans 1153, *entered into force* October 24, 1945.
3 International Covenant on Civil and Political Rights, G.A. res. 2200A (XXI), 21 U.N. GAOR Supp. (No. 16) at 52, U.N. Doc. A/6316 (1966), 999 U.N.T.S. 171, *entered into force* March 23, 1976.
4 International Covenant on Economic, Social and Cultural Rights, G.A. res. 2200A (XXI), 21 U.N.GAOR Supp. (No. 16) at 49, U.N. Doc. A/6316 (1966), 993 U.N.T.S. 3, *entered into force* January 3, 1976.
5 Convention on the Rights of the Child, G.A. res. 44/25, annex, 44 U.N. GAOR Supp. (No. 49) at 167, U.N. Doc. A/44/49 (1989), *entered into force* September 2, 1990.
6 Universal Declaration of Human Rights, G.A. res. 217A (III), U.N. Doc A/810 at 71 (1948).
7 Supplementary Convention on the Abolition of Slavery, the Slave Trade, and Institutions and Practices Similar to Slavery, 226 U.N.T.S. 3, *entered into force* April 30, 1957.
8 Convention for the Suppression of the Traffic in Persons and of the Exploitation of the Prostitution of Others, 96 U.N.T.S. 271, *entered into force* July 25, 1951.
9 Optional Protocol to the Convention on the Rights of the Child on the sale of Children, child prostitution and child pornography, G.A. Res. 54/263, Annex II,54 U.N. GAOR Supp. (No. 49) at 6, U.N. Doc. A/54/49, Vol. III (2000), *entered into force* January 18, 2002.
10 Optional Protocol to the Convention on the Rights of the Child on the involvement of children in armed conflicts, G.A. Res. 54/263, Annex I, 54 U.N. GAOR Supp. (No. 49) at 7, U.N. Doc. A/54/49, Vol. III (2000), *entered into force* February 12, 2002.
11 Convention Concerning the Prohibition and Immediate Action for the Elimination of the Worst Forms of Child Labor (ILO No. 182), 2133 U.N.T.S.161, *entered into force* November 19, 2000.
12 International Labour Organization Recommendation (No. 190) (1999). Concerning Worst Forms of Child Labour Convention, June 17, 1999, Geneva, Switzerland.
13 Convention concerning Forced or Compulsory Labour (ILO No. 29), 39 U.N.T.S. 55, *entered into force* May 1, 1932.
14 Convention concerning the Protection of Wages (ILO No. 95), *entered into force* September 24, 1952.
15 U.N. Comm. Hum. Rts. Res. 1990/68 ("Sale of Children"), U.N. Doc. E/CN.4/1990/94, at 145 (1990).
16 Constitution of the International Labour Organization, Oct. 9, 1946, 62 Stat. 3490, 15 U.N.T.S. 40, *entered into force* September 26, 1946. Available at http://training.itcilo.it/ILS/foa/library/constitution/iloconst_en.html#annex.

Chapter 8

Children's work and children's rights

Renata M. Coimbra Libório and
Silvia H. Koller

Introduction

Article 1 of the 1989 Convention on the Rights of the Child defines a child as being below the age of 18 years unless under law the age of majority is attained earlier [1]. The concept of age of majority, when adulthood is formally recognized and when a child ceases by law or convention to be a minor, is central to any discussion on rights. The rights of a child are not the same as the rights of an adult, and even while certain child rights may be fixed for the period of childhood, the importance of different rights may vary during that time. The right to protection for example is likely to have a particularly strong focus in younger children, whereas the right to participation is one that requires fuller expression as children grow.

It is well established that children are competent to exercise rights such as participation and self-expression [2]. The interpretation of those rights, however, is contextually and culturally defined [3]. Different social and cultural understandings of child development challenge any universal definition of interpretation of children's rights. In the context of children working, an understanding of the different meanings of work in children's lives is also closely tied to social and cultural interpretations of childhood. Furthermore, the speed at which children's capabilities evolve varies to some degree across different cultures [2].

This chapter examines children's rights in the framework of the United Nations Convention of the Rights of the Child with a focus on the rights to protection, provision and participation [1]. There is also some discussion on the rights to freedom of expression and freedom of association. This chapter also considers the linkages with other parts of the child labour model discussed throughout this book. In the context of rights these are most apparent with regard to social values.

The rights to protection, provision, and participation

The concept of childhood is socially and culturally constructed. Different groups, cultures, and societies establish their own definitions of what is meant by childhood and what is expected of children. Article 5 of the 1989 Convention notes that States parties must respect local custom and legal guardians in exercising the rights of the child. The Western consensus about the importance of school in children's lives, and the perspective of the child as an autonomous individual as required by the 1989 Convention does not, however, apply equally in all cultures. With regard to the 1989 Convention, Burr and Montgomery point out the contradiction between an acceptance of the validity of different cultural practices and any notion of universal rights [4]. This contradiction would, for example, challenge any concept of a universal minimum age for working.

Irrespective of any caveats with regard to the 1989 Convention, it is without doubt the best available tool for defining and guaranteeing children's rights. Both the 1989 Convention and the 1999 International Labour Organization (ILO) Convention no. 182 [5] state clearly that the practice of 'labour' by children breaches their human rights. The 1989 Convention establishes three sets of rights that have particular relevance to children working: the rights to protection, provision, and participation.

Protection

The right to protection concerns discrimination and punishment. Article 2 affirms that state parties shall 'take all appropriate measures to ensure that the child is protected against all forms of discrimination or punishment on the basis of the status, activities, expressed opinions, or the beliefs of the child's parents, legal guardians, or family members'.

Provision

The right to provision concerns the right to live in dignity and access to essential services. Article 3 of the 1989 Convention affirms that state parties shall undertake to ensure that children are afforded 'such protection and care as is necessary for his or her well-being, taking into account the rights and duties of his or her parents, legal guardians, or other individuals legally responsible for him or her, and, to this end, shall take all appropriate legislative and administrative measures'. Furthermore, 'State parties shall ensure that the institutions, service and facilities responsible for the care or protection of children shall conform with standards established by competent authorities...'

Participation

The right to participation concerns the recognition of children's rights to have an input into decisions related to their well-being, freedom of expression, freedom of thought, meet peacefully and to form their own associations.

Article 12 of the 1989 Convention states that state parties are responsible for assuring that a 'child who is capable of forming his or her own views [has] the right to express those views freely in all matters affecting the child, the views of the child being given due weight in accordance with the age and maturity of the child'. Article 12 places this right in the particular context of 'judicial and administrative proceedings affecting the child… either directly or through a representative…'.

Further definition of this right to participation is given in subsequent Articles. Article 13 states that 'The child shall have the right to freedom of expression…' while Article 14 states that 'State parties shall respect the rights and duties of the child to freedom of thought, conscience and religion… in a manner consistent with the evolving capacities of the child'. Article 15 recognizes the child's right to 'freedom of association and peaceful assembly'.

Rights in reality

Guaranteeing the rights to provision and protection presents a challenge especially to less economically developed countries. The right to participation has been difficult to assure in many societies, perhaps more so in some economically developed countries.

Protection and provision are closely connected, and for a variety of reasons are often neglected or incompletely implemented. A measure of social consensus, infrastructure, and support is needed to assure the rights to protection and provision [6]. A failure to provide basic needs such as food, shelter, and education creates a violation of these basic rights. However, in many agricultural communities, on the streets of large cities, and in some industrial communities there is a lack of such infrastructure, which combined with pressing economic circumstances means that children have to work in order to survive.

As a result of illness or even death in a parent, children themselves may become responsible for the maintenance of their family, especially younger siblings. Thrust prematurely into an adult role, these children face physical, psychological, and developmental risks. The rights of these children to protection and provision are clearly incompatible with their labour activities and as such are violated.

Globally, many families, communities, and governments have not been able to offer children access to 'institutions, services and facilities' as indicated in Article 3 that will guarantee their rights to protection and provision. In such circumstances children may find alternative protection and provision in activities that have a negative effect on their health and development. At one extreme children have found protection and provision for their basic needs by joining army groups, even when a particular conflict has resulted in the death of their family members and the disappearance of their communities [7].

In other pressing social and economic circumstances, children have taken to the streets to engage in a variety of informal work. The commercial sexual exploitation of children has also brought children a degree of provision that they may have deemed essential for survival [8, 9].

The responsibility of guaranteeing children's rights to provision and protection falls upon adults. These rights require a commitment from families and communities, a wider civil society; health, educational, and welfare professionals, and most of all a political commitment from national and international governments. Implementing children's rights to provision and protection requires consideration of a wide range of potential strategies such as improving education and health facilities as well as living conditions. It may also, where appropriate, involve providing age-appropriate employment opportunities.

While millions of children around the world continue to face extreme poverty, and consequently become involved in harmful labour activities in order to obtain food, shelter and resources for themselves and often their families, their rights to protection and provision will remain breached. Inadequate family income, a lack of social support and ineffective public policies keep children working [10, 11].

The right to participation is quite distinct from the rights to provision and protection and concerns the many forms of involvement and engagement. It has been described as the most difficult of children's rights to ensure, especially if governments, civil society, and institutions do not work together [4, 12]. Growing up in a supportive family environment is considered the ideal for the child and the family offers the optimum context in which to ensure children's welfare and rights [13]. The idea of 'belonging' to a family does have limits – a child belongs to her/his family, but as a member, not as property.

According to Kirby and Woodhead, the concept of children's participation encompasses a 'positive image of inclusion, engagement and consensus' and their participation should encompass a range of settings such as health programmes, school projects, and children's clubs [14]. Not all child participation is, however, active, meaningful, or constructive. Whereas the rights to protection and provision stem from adults; to be meaningful, the right to participation has to come from children. It has been observed that in some cases children's participation has become adult-centric and even imposed by adults upon children [15].

Burr and Montgomery identify two different approaches to securing children's rights: the protectionist and the participatory [4]. With protectionism, children are viewed as needing adult protection and help. Adults make decisions on behalf of children. The participatory approach states that children need to be empowered to make decisions on their own behalf. In part, these two approaches can be explained on the basis of age and competence. However, there is no chronological age when all children achieve the same level of competence, and that to a degree, competence is dependent on cultural and social context.

The influence of child work on children's rights

With regard to children working, the right to participation and the context within which it is played out illustrates one of the paradoxes in implementing the different rights of children. In certain situations it would appear that even when work carries with it considerable potential and actual health hazards, children and their communities argue strongly for their right to continue working in these circumstances. This paradox is considered in more detail in the case study of coco babaçu workers in North East Brazil later in this book.

Work in itself may not necessarily be an infringement on children's rights. Some children who work and go to school are in good health, and have family and community support. Moreover, through their work activity they express a meaning in their lives and a sense of self-worth. Many studies have concluded that certain types of work, in specific conditions are positive experiences for children [16–20]. Positive outcomes include increased self esteem, self efficacy, and identity development.

Even in situations of intolerable working conditions, an emerging literature suggests that there may be some positive experiences. For example, young street workers [9, 21] and child soldiers [7] have been shown to demonstrate considerable resilience. Resilience has been defined as the positive aspects of development that are related to the capacity of negotiate for resources to sustain well-being [22]. It appears that some children may be able to endure extreme adverse labour conditions and later successfully return to more normal circumstances. Of course, this in no way justifies such types of labour but it does indicate that there may be some hope for children living in such severe conditions. It should be emphasized that this is not a generalization of all children working in intolerable conditions, and in fact in the case of child soldiers, this view is in direct conflict with what has been documented with regard to the development of psychiatric disorders among some adult soldiers, thus calling into question the validity of the research findings on children.

Nevertheless, as to Woodhead notes, it is not simply a question of the type of work but also a question of the values attributed to work by the family and community which influence the feelings of self-worth and self-esteem experienced by children [23]. When work activity is respected and valued, and it is not stigmatized, these feelings increase significantly. In contrast when families or communities are ashamed of children's work, no such positive feelings are experienced by children.

Researchers and policy makers in the field of child labour need therefore to be responsive to children's voices and take this into account in the design of research and of services [14, 24–26]. They need to take account of diverse cultures, different understandings of gender roles, and the development of identity, responsibility, agency, and autonomy. Some authors have questioned the value of a universal minimum-age approach on child labour (ILO Convention no. 138) suggesting that there is insufficient empirical evidence that children benefit from being withdrawn or excluded from work and some evidence to question it. They stress the importance of understanding the impact of work on working children's lives and suggest that there should be more contextualization of the idea of a minimum-age, rather than a universal policy [27].

That said, children's work is often the result of abusive and exploitative power relationships. However, where children's work is truly a 'choice', the right to work, as has been stated by some social movements of working children, can be seen as an expression of children's rights to participate. Children's agency and autonomy are important components of meaningful participation. Since the first such movement arose in 1976, in several Latin American, Asian, and African countries working children's organizations have taken action to protect working children [28, 29, 30].

Some of these movements are considered to be good examples of how children's rights to protection, provision, and participation can be ensured. Many of these movements also address the role of citizenship. Children's involvement is an expression of their right to actively participate, politically and economically, in the decisions in their community and the wider society [29]. Their participation is also an expression of their rights to freedom of expression and association. The possibility of children establishing their own rights is stressed in many organizations such as the African Movement of Working Children and Youth [28], the Movimiento de Ninos y Ninas Trabajadores Hijos de Obreros Cristianos [31], Ninos y Adolescentes Trabajadores [32] and the International Movement of Working Children [33].

Liebel (2006) has examined the main objectives of such movements around the world and found common themes: campaigns for guaranteed quality education and health care; a crusade against discrimination, poverty, violence, and exploitation; demands for work with dignity; and action to have children's labour movements formally recognized with representation at national and international level protected by legislation [29]. There is some evidence that a significant impact has resulted from such participation.

In some countries there have been improvements in the living conditions of working children as well as solidarity among children. Some organizations have succeeded in developing training courses in order that children may be better qualified and improve their future employment prospects. There is also evidence of some impact on legislation, as has occurred in Brazil and Peru. These efforts have resulted in a decrease of discrimination, more respectful treatment by the police, improved health services, and support from the research community [25]. It is important to understand, however, that these movements do not represent an alternative to, or a substitute for, the role required of civil society and government, and many working children across the poorer parts of the world still face exploitation and a violation of their rights on a daily basis.

Conclusions

The 1989 Convention on the Rights of the Child represents an important step in guaranteeing the rights of children. However, the rights to protection, provision, and participation, and to freedom of expression and association are understood differently in different societies in accordance with social and cultural perspectives. One of the challenges of ensuring that these rights are guaranteed is creating a wider understanding of the different perspectives on children, childhood, and the roles of children, families, and communities with regard to work and early development.

Most children around the world meet their needs to protection and provision through their families and communities. In situations where families and communities appear to fail, this may be simply a reflection of the failure of national institutions and international support. Children are sometimes pushed into very hazardous occupations in an effort to seek some protection and to provide for their and sometimes others' basic needs.

It is evident that children need to be protected and to be provided for and that this should come from adults. In order to ensure the right of participation, even when this appears to conflict with other rights, adults must value children's agency. The development of a positive identity and feelings of pride by children is not only possible through relationships with parents and other responsible adults. Children's participation may at times appear to be in conflict with their rights to protection and provision. This raises the question of a hierarchy of rights, which is not suggested in the Convention on the Rights of the Child, but merits further consideration.

Even if all child work were eliminated, it is not clear that the rights of children would be assured. There is insufficient research into the ways in which work diminishes the long-term ability of a child to participate in society through the loss of educational opportunities. All those concerned with implementing universal children's rights need to recognize that what constitutes full and appropriate implementation will vary depending on the circumstances of different families and communities.

References

1 United Nations (UN) (1990). Convention on the rights of the child. Available at http://www2.ohchr.org/english/law/pdf/crc.pdf (accessed 10 May 2008).

2 Daiute C (2008). The rights of children, the rights of nations: Developmental theory and the politics of children's rights. *Journal of Social Issues*, **64**(4):701–23.

3 Rogers WS (2003). What is a child? In Woodhead M, Montgomery H (eds), *Understanding Childhood: An Interdisciplinary Approach*, pp. 1–43. The Open University, Wiley & Sons, UK.

4 Burr R, Montgomery H (2003). Children and rights. In Woodhead M, Montgomery H (eds), *Understanding Childhood: An Interdisciplinary Approach*, pp. 135–78. The Open University, Wiley & Sons, UK.

5 International Labour Organizations (ILO) (2002). Eliminating the worst forms of child labour: A practical guide to ILO Convention no. 182. Available at http://www.ilocarib.org.tt/childlabour/library/ParliamentaryHandbook.pdf (accessed 12 June 2008).

6 Soares NF (2005). Os direitos das crianças nas encruzilhadas da proteção e da participação. Available at http://www.periodicos.ufsc.br/index.php/zeroseis/article/viewFile/2100/1780 (accessed 15 February 2008].

7 Cortes L, Buchanan MJ (2007). The experience of Columbian child soldiers from a resilience perspective. *International Journal for the Advancement of Counselling*, **29**(1):43–55.

8 Invernizzi A (2003). Street working children and adolescents in Lima – work as an agent of socialization. *Childhood*, **10**(3):319–41.

9 Perez-Carreon JG (2006). *Street work girls in Mexico City: Pathways to resilience in an adverse world.* Unpublished doctoral dissertation, The University of Texas, Austin, Texas, USA.

10 Cruz MNA and Assuncao AA (2008). Estrutura e Organizacao do trabalho infantil em situacao de rua em Belo Horizonte, MG, Brasil. *Saude Soc Sao Paulo*, **17**(1):131–42.

11 Jacquemin MY (2004). Children's domestic work in Abidjan, Cote D'Ivoire: The petites bonnes have the floor. *Childhood*, **11**(3):383–97.

12 Pinto M, Sarmento MJ (eds). (1997). *As crianças, contextos e identidades.* Braga, Portugal: Universidade do Minho Press.

13 Koller SH, De Antoni C (2004). Violência intrafamiliar: uma visão ecológica. In Koller SH (ed.), *Ecologia do Desenvolvimento Humano: Pesquisa e Intervenção no Brasil.* São Paulo, SP, Brasil: Casa do Psicólogo.

14 Kirby P, Woodhead M (2003). Children's participation in society. In Montgomery H, Burr R,Woodhead M (eds), *Changing Childhoods: Local and Global*, pp. 233–72. The Open University: Wiley & Sons, UK.

15 United Nations (UN) (2003). The state of the world's children. Available at http://www.unicef.org/sowc03/contents/pdf/SOWC03-eng.pdf (accessed 20 February 2009).

16 Amazarray M, Thome L, Poletto M, and Koller S (2007). Perspectivas acerca do trabalho infant-juvenil: ideologias, subjectividade e saude do trabalhador. *Laboreal*, **III**(2):22–8.

17 Bey M (2003). The Mexican child: From work with the family to paid employment. *Childhood*, **10**(3):287–99.

18 Hugerland B, Liebel M, Lisecke A, Wihstutz A (2007). Paths to participatory autonomy: The meanings of work for children in Germany. *Childhood*, **14**(2):257–77.

19 Rubenson B (2005). *Working children's experience and their right to health and Well*-being. Stockholm, Sweden: Karolinska University Press.

20 Woodhead M, Montgomery H (2004). *Understanding Childhood: An Interdisciplinary Approach*. The Open University: Wiley & Sons, UK.

21 Kidd S, Shahar G (2008). Resilience in homeless youth: The key role of self-esteem. *American Journal of Orthopsychiatry*, **78**(2):163–72.

22 Ungar M (2008). Resilience across cultures. *British Journal of Social Work*, **38**(2): 218–35.

23 Woodhead M (2004). Psychosocial impacts of child work: A framework for research, monitoring and intervention. *The International Journal of Children's Rights*, **12**: 321–77.

24 Leonard M (2004). Children's views on children's right to work: Reflections from Belfast. *Childhood*, **11**(1):45–61.

25 Liebel M (2003).Working children as social subjects. *Childhood*, **10**(3):265–85.

26 Woodhead M (1999). Combating child labour: Listen to what children say. *Childhood* **6**(1):27–49.

27 Bourdillon MFC, White B, and Myers WE (2009). Re-assessing minimum-age standards for children's work. *International Journal of Sociology and Social Policy*, **29**(3/4):106.

28 Liebel M (2004). *A will of their own – cross cultural perspectives on working children*. Chicago: Zed Books.

29 Liebel M (2006). Ciudadanía desde abajo: Los movimientos sociales de niños trabajadores. Paper presented at Ciclo de Conferencias: Sociologia da Infancia, University of Minho, Portugal.

30 Movimiento Latinoamericano y del Caribe de Niños/as y Adolescentes Trabajadores, 2008 *Declaración de Cachipay*. Available at http://molacnats.org/index.php?option=com_content&task=view&id=74&Itemid=81 (accessed 15 December 2008).

31 Movimiento de Adolescentes y Ninos Trabajadores Hijos de Obreros Cristianos. Nuestra historia. Available at http://www.manthocperu.org/contenido/index.php?option=com_content&task=view&id=24&Itemid=47 (accessed 30 November 2008).

32 Los niños, niñas y adolescentes trabajadores (NATs). Available at http://www.accionporlosninos.org.pe/pdfs/pccnt.pdf (accessed October 2008).

33 The International Working Children Movement (1996). Available at http://www.workingchild.org/prota2.htm (accessed 15 December 2008).

Chapter 9

Understanding the health effects of child labour

David L. Parker, Anaclaudia G. Fassa, and Thomas J. Scanlon

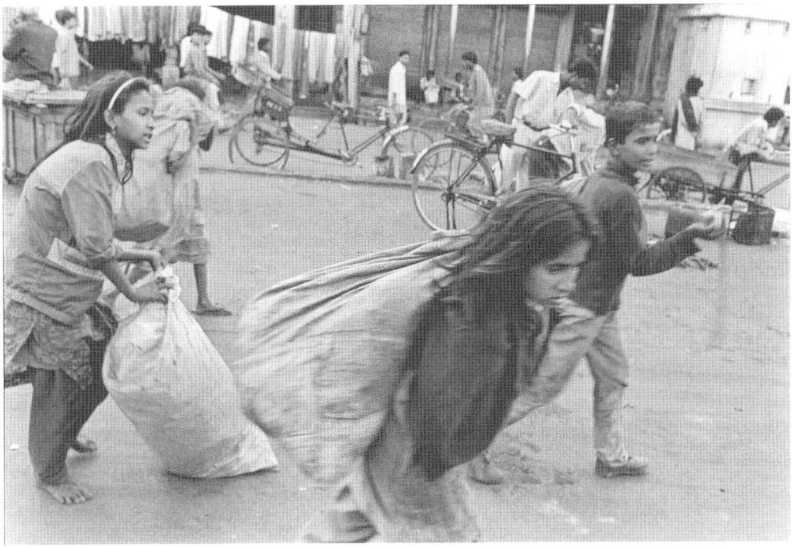

Garbage pickers, Nepal

Introduction

Child work is a continuum, and there is no clear demarcation of when work moves from a positive experience to a harmful one. In spite of the risks posed by many forms of work, for large numbers of children, the alternative to work may be hunger or other adverse outcomes. This chapter describes the health effects of children's work and the impact of this work on the communities in which they live. The focus of this chapter is child labour and hazardous work as defined by the International Labour Organization (ILO).[1] For the purpose of simplicity, these are collectively referred to herein as child labour. The chapter follows the public health model of child labour referred to throughout this book and considers both the direct health effects on the individual and the broader social environment that facilitates or impairs the health and well-being of individuals and communities.

In general, there is a dearth of literature with regard to the health effects of child labour on children and communities. The health impacts discussed in this section have therefore been selected not on the basis of presenting a comprehensive review of what has been written, but rather as examples of the range of adverse health effects experienced by child labourers and to illustrate the gaps in existing knowledge. As such, it provides guidance to readers with regard to how to understand the scope of the effects of work on the health of children as well as how hazards may impact well-being within communities.

Following this introduction, subsequent chapters illustrate specific health problems; HIV/AIDS, lead poisoning, pesticide toxicity, silicotuberculosis, injuries, and psychosocial and developmental problems. While at times there are potential health benefits associated with some child work such as improved nutrition and higher levels of self-esteem, these chapters when taken together suggest that the adverse health effects associated with child labour considerably outweigh the benefits and that they are greater than is generally considered in the current literature.

This introductory chapter is divided into three parts. First, it examines the difficulties in determining the impact of child labour on health. Second, it describes approaches which can help in understanding the impact of child labour. Third, it presents examples of the impact of child labour on the health of children, families, and communities and how these impacts might be more effectively measured.

[1] Not all work done by children should be classified as child labour that should be targeted for elimination. Children's or adolescents' participation in work that does not affect their health and personal development or interfere with their schooling is generally regarded as being something positive. This includes activities such as helping their parents around the home, assisting in a family business, or earning pocket money outside school hours and during school holidays. These kinds of activities may contribute to children's development and to the welfare of their families; they provide them with skills and experience and help to prepare them to be productive members of society during their adult life.

See Chapter 2 for a full discussion on child work and child labour definitions.

Difficulties in determining the impact of child labour on health

Considerable resources and rigorous study design are required in order to estimate the impact of child labour on health [1]. However, rigorous study design is not easy even when resources are available. Defining and measuring the impact of work on health and communities may be difficult for multiple reasons, as detailed below.

Hidden and illegal work

Attempts to understand the health impact of hidden and illegal work are fraught with problems [1]. For example, it is virtually impossible to study the health impact on children held in forced and bonded labour. The International Labour Office notes, 'At least 12.3 million people around the world are trapped in forced labour. Forced labour takes different forms, including debt bondage, trafficking and other forms of modern slavery' [2].

Defining populations at risk

Studies often employ a broad definition of child labour. This may result in a heterogeneous group of workers and work conditions, and the adverse effects from specific occupations (e.g. brick making) may be diluted. This is especially true if harmful work is found much less often than work which is not harmful. While the overall well-being of a community may be high, social disparities and related working conditions disproportionately affect some segments of societies. For example, in some instances working children may be better nourished than non-working children, however, it is unlikely that children working in garbage dumps would be afforded the benefits that might accrue to children working in a protected environment.

As is discussed in the social values section of this book, there is strong evidence that harmful work is not uniformly distributed across all social groups or by gender. It is equally true that the risk of harm is not uniformly spread throughout different occupations and sectors of the economy. There is a need to more clearly define risk within sub-populations [3].

Healthy worker effect

The adverse effects of some types of work may be underestimated because of selection bias in what is referred to as the 'healthy worker' effect. Children may be selected for work because they are healthier than their peers, and they may leave work as a result of illness or injury. However, the status of injured child workers may place them at risk in other types of employment. An inverse effect may also apply, and the healthiest children with the greatest potential may be selected for a school education [4].

Latency

Latency refers to the time period between the onset of exposure and the onset of disease. Numerous illnesses are preceded by a long latency period. This may lead to attributing illness to a later period in life, and failure to properly attribute work as causal. For most exposures, cancers are preceded by a latency period of 20 or more years. Few cancers are specific to work exposures and it is difficult to attribute most cancers to specific places or times of work. Other illnesses, such as dust-related lung diseases (e.g. pneumoconiosis) may also be preceded by a long latency period. It is well established that most cases of silicosis have a latency period of at least 10–20 years. Thus children may not experience illness until they are young adults.

Misdiagnosis and under-recognition of problems

Illness may be under-recognized or misdiagnosed. Work-related problems may go unrecognized and their aetiology attributed to the wrong cause. Job-specific hazards are difficult to identify. For example, a wide range of exposures such as mineral and organic dusts, isocyanates, and acute chemical exposures cause or exacerbate asthma [5]. Work-related asthma, however, is symptomatically identical to asthma of other causes. Among adults, 18–25% of asthma cases are caused by or worsened from work [6].

Difficulty in measuring developmental changes

Developmental changes are difficult to measure even if the effects of a toxin are well established. Neurotoxicity and problems related to organ development have been well documented for pharmaceutical agents, heavy metals including lead, mercury, cadmium, and arsenic, as well as pesticides, and nicotine. Neurotoxicity can cause impaired intellectual development, behavioural problems, and aberrations of brain growth and development. These changes are complex to evaluate and are influenced by education, nutritional status, pre-natal care, and substance abuse, among others [7, 8].

Difficulty in measuring psychosocial effects

As is discussed later in this book, there is little evidence on the effects of work on the psychosocial well-being of working children. There is a lack of valid and reliable tools to measure psychosocial effects in different cultures. It has, however, been well recognised for some time that working children are vulnerable to abuse and exploitation and as such are at risk of serious adverse psychosocial effects [9].

Inter-generational harm

Harm may be transmitted across generations. This may be secondary to environmental contamination or toxins crossing the placental barrier. The impact of some environmental exposures on the foetus is well-documented. Heavy metals, especially lead, cadmium, mercury, and pesticides affect fetal development [10, 11].

Congenital malformations or other disabilities may occur in the children of pregnant workers exposed to toxins. For example, a teenage woman engaged in the extraction of gold using mercury is susceptible to harm to herself as well as her children should she become pregnant. Potential intergenerational effects of toxic substances may mean that children begin life with lower intelligence or other neuro-cognitive changes placing them at risk of failure in school and early entry into the workforce [8].

Co-morbidity

There is substantial evidence that adverse socio-economic conditions will adversely affect the health of children and adults [12]. Any evaluation of the impact of work-related exposures needs to take into account the baseline health of exposed individuals. The effect of work and environmental exposures in combination with poor health complicates an understanding of the impact of work on the current and future health of children and communities, emphasizing the need for a complex analytical approach as described in the following paragraphs.

Approaches which can help in understanding the impact of child labour

Child labour data would be substantially improved by increasing the scope of global surveillance programmes related to child labour. Surveillance data might include specific illnesses such as silicosis, pesticide toxicity, or traumatic injury. The expansion of national data would facilitate the use of international and national resources.

A number of study designs may be used to examine the long-term health effects of work. Ideally, studies would be conducted in different settings around the world. They should address possible confounding and interacting variables, as well as include control groups with non-workers, workers in other occupations, and workers with different degrees of exposure in order to avoid selection bias. However, these studies are very difficult to undertake in the circumstances of child labour.

Child labour-specific studies

While increasing in number, there are few studies of working children that describe the effects of different work conditions and exposures on child growth, development, and well-being. This reflects the practical difficulties in both undertaking research in child labour settings and measuring work hazards and related illnesses.

In general, studies are based on small sample sizes. Nevertheless, they provide useful evidence of the impact of work on child health. For example, a study of crafts workers in Morocco indicated substantial health problems though it failed to identify the aetiology of the problems [13]. A cross-sectional study of solvent exposures in 300 children in Lebanon aged 10–17 years provided evidence of solvent toxicity. The authors noted, 'Memory and motor dexterity appear to be particularly affected in solvent-exposed working children. These effects are likely to have implications for the capacity of the exposed children to respond to new demands and to learn new information' [14].

Other studies focus on more generalized effects rather than specific hazards. Particularly common are studies evaluating the impact of work on education. For example, Teixeira *et al.* examined the impact of adolescent work on sleep patterns and academic performance. They reported that working students may have their learning ability negatively affected by being tired and sleepy [15]. A separate study of working children also reported problems with academic performance because of sleep deprivation [16].

Given the difficulties in undertaking studies of the health effects of children's work and the resultant relative lack of data, other means have to be sought to estimate the impact of work on children. These include studies of toxic exposure to children from non-work related causes and occupational health studies of adults.

Studies of non-working children

One way of estimating the health impacts of child labour is through epidemiological studies of the effects of environmental exposures in non-working children. This may be done using scientific studies that address chemical exposures, toxicology, pharmacology, and metabolism among infants and children. Studies exist for a wide range of substances such as heavy metals, pesticides, dioxins, and hormonally active compounds. In a subsequent chapter, lead is presented as an example as to how data of non-working children may be used to evaluate the impact of work on children.

Wigle discusses a wide range of studies on the impact of environmental contaminants on children. For example, polyhalogenated aromatic hydrocarbons (PHAHs), a group of common industrial toxins, have been linked to severe acne (chloracne). Long-term studies of numerous substances have shown problems with developmental delays, abnormal behaviours, and abnormal growth patterns [17].

Asthma provides another important example of the impact of a variety of toxins on health. A wide range of environmental agents can cause or exacerbate asthma among children. These include environmental tobacco smoke, home use of a gas stove for heat, pets, or exposure to farm animals [17]. In developing nations, studies of children exposed to smoke from wood cooking stoves have shown a substantially increased risk of developing symptoms of asthma [18]. Acute respiratory infection in children, one of the chief causes of infant and childhood mortality, has been associated with household smoke exposures [19].

Studies of adults

Studies of adult workers provide important data on the impact of work on health and well-being. These findings can be extrapolated to the potential impact of similar work on the health and well-being of children and communities. For a number of reasons, however, the extrapolation of adult data to children may under-estimate the extent of harm to child labourers.

Recent research indicates that there is a complex relationship between age at the time of exposure and outcome. There are critical periods during development when different regions of the brain, lungs, gastro-intestinal tract, and other organs are highly susceptible to harm [5, 20]. Significant organ development occurs through adolescence and into early adulthood. For example, the endocrine system is an important target for toxicants, particularly during adolescence, altering the hormonal balance and/or its feedback loops, and has negative effects on development and sexual maturation [8, 21]. These kinds of effects are difficult to predict because different organs and organ systems mature at different rates and at different times of life [22].

Relative to their weight, children have a larger surface area increasing the risk of trans-cutaneous absorption of toxins. The United States Agency for Toxic Substances and Disease Registries (ATSDR) notes that in similar environments, children may have greater exposures than adults, 'Pound for pound of body weight, children drink more water, eat more food, and breathe more air than adults' and 'in some instances, children are less able than adults to detoxify chemicals and are thus more vulnerable' [23].

Physical trauma and heat exposure are two other examples of the differential effect of age on outcome. Adolescents are at risk of injury to ligaments and to bone-growth plates. This is especially true during periods of rapid growth. Injuries to growth plates may have long-term consequences such as unequal limb length. Where heat exposure is a hazard (e.g. farming, brick kilns), the greater surface area-to-body mass ratio of children will result in greater heat gain from the environment on a hot day and greater heat loss to the environment on a cold day [24].

The impact of children's work on health of children, families, and communities

There is no accepted and simple way to classify the effects of child labour on the health of children and communities [25–27]. The effects of job-related hazards are often considered in terms of chemical, biological, and physical agents, and their impact on health. Hazards are also discussed with regard to job tasks within specific sectors (e.g. brick making) in which children work [25, 28].

Following these models, job hazards are divided into biological (e.g. insects, plants, organic dusts), chemical (e.g. mercury, lead), physical (e.g. heavy weight, ergonomic), and psychosocial (e.g. long hours, physical abuse) hazards. Most of these categories may be further subdivided into those leading to acute-onset harm (e.g. injury, pesticide poisoning) and chronic-illness including developmental problems [25, 27, 28]. In some instances, they may also result in broader health problems within the community.

There is no clear point when an outcome changes from acute to chronic. The nature of child labour is that several hazards will co-exist. Hazards rarely exist in isolation from each other, and many exposures result in both acute and chronic illness (e.g. lead, mercury). The discussion of occupational exposures and acute and chronic health outcomes on individuals, families, and communities outlined below is not encompassing. However, it offers a starting point for understanding the potential adverse health effects of work on individuals and communities.

The distinction between acute and latent harm is difficult to apply to community health. Perhaps the most frequent cause of acute contamination is from pesticides. For example, aerial spraying may result in community contamination [29]. Long-term contamination may occur both within and around the workplace. For example, mercury is often used to extract gold. As the gold–mercury amalgam is heated, the mercury contaminates the ambient environment.

Table 9.1 shows the impact of selected occupations and related hazardous exposures on the health of individual children and the community. While a discussion of occupational exposures and acute and chronic health outcomes on individuals and communities as outlined in the table below is not all encompassing, it offers a starting point for the examination of the potential adverse health effects of work on individuals and communities.

Table 9.1 The impact of a sample of work-related exposures on the health of individuals and the community

Sample occupations	Hazardous exposure*	Individual acute effect	Individual latent or chronic effect	Community effects	Selected references
Gold mining	Mining dusts Mercury	Rare Acute toxicity	Silicosis Microcephaly, mental impairment	Environmental contamination from waste and mercury	[30] See chapter on silico-tuberculosis in this volume
Garbage picking	Vermin Contaminated water Machinery	Infectious diseases Injuries	Chronic parasitic diseases	Water and other environmental contamination	[31, 32]
Brick making	Silica dust Air pollution	Rare Asthma, acute bronchial injury	Silicosis Asthma	Dust Air pollution from brick kilns	[33, 34]
Leather tanning	Anthrax Heavy metals	Acute anthrax Acute toxicity, dermatitis	Chronic toxicity from heavy metals	Environmental contamination from effluent	[35–37]
Carpet weaving	Dusts, fibres Repetitive work Dim lighting Abusive work	Asthma, dermatitis Tendonitis, eye strain Failure to thrive	Asthma Osteoarthritis Failure to thrive Post-traumatic stress	Effluent from dying	[38,39] [40] [41]
Shoe shining	Exhaust from cars Contamination of polish Street violence	Lead Lead, gasoline Sexual violence	Chronic toxicity from heavy metals Sexually transmitted disease	Air pollution	[42]
Tobacco picking	Nicotine, pesticides Sun exposure	Nicotine poisoning, pesticide toxicity Sun burn	 Skin cancer	Pesticide contamination	[43, 44]

* This is **not** a complete listing of hazardous exposures for each type of work. Rather, these are examples to illustrate the different health effects that may result from the work commonly done by children.

As seen in Table 9.1, most exposures have both an acute and a latent effect on the individual as well as on the surrounding community. Some of these effects have been well studied (e.g. mercury contamination of the ambient environment). However, others go largely unnoticed (e.g. effluent from carpet dyes, air pollution from brick kilns). For example, while no studies were found of asthma among children who manufacture bricks, it is likely that asthma is a consequence of heavy air pollution. Children have no chance of escaping this pollution because they both live and work within the contaminated environment.

Physical hazards

Acute effects

The epidemiological literature illustrates the acute harm faced by working children and adolescents. In the United States, where adolescents work in relatively protected environments, injury represents an ongoing problem. In the agricultural sector, there are frequent reports of children and youth being seriously injured or killed at work [45].

Studies conducted in the United States of teenage workers have generally shown a substantially increased risk of injury when compared to their adult peers. For example, workers aged 19 years and under experience a significantly greater proportion of fatalities due to violence in the retail trades and construction trades than their counterparts in other industries [46–49].

It is not surprising that the incidence of injury is higher for working youth than adults. Machinery, equipment, and tools are designed for adult use. Mismatches between a child or adolescent's size and the equipment used increase the risk of fatigue, injuries, and musculoskeletal problems. This raises concerns about the operation of machinery by children and adolescents [45, 50, 51].

There are obvious risks from many occupations such as brick making, mining, scavenging garbage, and other work. 'Brick workers and miners carry heavy loads and are exposed to high levels of dust. Garbage scavengers work around heavy machinery, including trucks and bulldozers, and children climb on top of moving trucks. Trucks may empty their contents indiscriminately on or near children and adults. Spontaneous combustion causes constant small fires, and occasionally landslides occur [52].

Chronic effects

In the course of compiling this book, few studies documenting the long-term effects of work injury on children were identified. Parker *et al.* note problems with acute traumatic injury causing herniated inter-vertebral discs secondary to heavy lifting [53]. These injuries are likely to lead to ongoing disability.

Children may be engaged in repetitive work that involves high force and awkward postures such as making bricks or crushing rock. Although little research has focused on ergonomic stressors to children and adolescents, ergonomic stressors are likely to be an important cause of chronic injury [54]. Lee discusses the mismatching of child and adolescent workers to specific job-related tasks in a case study included in this in volume.

Chemical hazards

Acute effects

Acute toxic exposures to child and adolescent workers are poorly documented. Exposures include heavy metals, pesticides, solvents, unknown contaminants in waste, and a host of other agents found in poorly controlled agricultural and industrial environments.

For example, children working in tobacco fields are susceptible to the effects of nicotine and develop acute nicotine poisoning, known as green tobacco sickness. The illness is characterized by nausea, vomiting, headaches, and muscle weakness. Child and adolescent workers are at an increased risk of developing this illness compared with their more experienced peers who develop nicotine tolerance [55].

Tobacco workers are also exposed to the uncontrolled use of pesticides. A study of tobacco workers in Pakistan identified pesticide toxicity in 56% of farmers (n=61 out of 108). The authors noted, 'Most farmers had little knowledge about the safety measures', and that there was a 'casual attitude and unsatisfactory safety practices with regard to the use of basic protective equipments during pesticide applications on the tobacco crop' [43].

Chronic effects

No studies were found that examine the long-term effects of occupational chemical exposures to children. However, non-occupational studies of the impact of many substances on the health of children do exist. Perhaps the best studied of these is lead. As described more fully elsewhere in this volume, children absorb lead more than adults and are at significantly more risk of developing irreversible neurological damage. Studies have also been conducted on the impact of mercury and carbon monoxide. Both are common occupational exposures. Data indicate an impact of both substances on early growth and development. These substances are also well-documented reproductive hazards [55].

Biological hazards

Acute effects

Children may be exposed to a wide array of biological hazards in a number of occupations. Among garbage workers, puncture wounds are common and may result in tetanus [56, 57]. A survey of 740 scavenger children in Cambodia found common tropical diseases such as malaria and infections as well as a range of debilitating conditions, from fevers to body pains of undefined origins [58].

In agriculture, exposures include natural poisons such as nicotine [55], venomous bites and stings [53], and vector-borne disease such as malaria, dengue, or other acute illnesses. These are not usually considered work-related problems, and there is no documentation that records them as such.

Chronic effects

Silicotuberculosis is discussed in more detail elsewhere in this book. Silicosis caused by exposure to dust found in many common occupations such as brickwork, stone crushing, and mining is often found in tandem with tuberculosis. Common acute illnesses that are likely to affect workers due to poor sanitation may become chronic. Examples include amoebiasis, giardia, salmonella, or other illnesses resulting from poor sanitation and unacceptable food quality.

Psychosocial hazards

Many abusive practices arise in the workplace. These include long hours, poor housing and sanitation, lack of potable water, gender discrimination, violence, and low wages [47, 60]. There has been some study of the effect of long hours on well-being and academic achievement. However, in general, these problems are not well described with regard to their impact on the health and well-being of child and adolescent workers and the communities in which they live.

The importance of worker rights, and the rights of immigrant, migrant, and non-citizens should not be overlooked in any analysis of the effects of work on children. These populations are frequently undercounted, and their rights subject to abuse. Many live in fear of deportation. Human Rights Watch points to the lack of sanitary facilities, hand washing facilities, and potable water for adolescent migrant workers in the United States. They also note problems with wage fraud and the sexual harassment of girls [61].

Domestic workers are largely hidden from public view and are the frequent victims of violence [62]. In some countries, labour laws are not applied to domestic workers who are considered to be of little social value. Women may be held in near captivity because their wages are kept in order to pay for their cost of travel to and lodging within their place of work [63].

While this may seem to be a small population, Weissbrodt points out that 3% of the world's population currently reside in a nation other than that in which they were born. He notes, 'The pressure to be competitive encourages many enterprises to employ cheap and often irregular migrant workers in sectors such as agriculture, garment manufacturing, domestic service and the sex industry' [64]. All these industries are frequent employers of children.

Community effects

Community health is an important aspect of the model on child labour discussed in this book. Many contaminants (e.g. pesticides, lead, and mercury) are dispersed into the ambient environment causing contamination of the home, water supplies, and land. This wider impact points to the importance of understanding the ambient and home environment in addition to trying to understand the effects of work on health.

The widespread contamination of communities from mining and industrial effluents may harm entire ecosystems and result in the displacement of communities as well as causing toxicity in individuals [65]. In the case of gold mining, the waste materials result in both immediate toxicity as well as secondary environmental contamination [66].

Burning materials are a common source of indoor and community-wide pollution. Smoke from brick kilns is likely to contribute to indoor air pollution as a cause of asthma. Approximately 50% of the world's population relies on some type of biomass as a fuel [67].

While work may impact community health, the corollary, community illness may impact the need for children to work. For example, HIV and AIDS have had an enormous impact on child labour both as a cause and a consequence. HIV and AIDS have decimated the adult population of sub-Saharan Africa. In the absence of adult workers and caregivers, children have by necessity, undertaken work typically occupied by adults. This impact has been mediated through its effects on families, communities, and national economies. This is explored more fully later in this book.

Educational attainment is another important community-based outcome. Children who live in homes where the parents, particularly the mothers, are better educated are more likely to go to school and stay in school longer. For children who live in homes where their parents received little or no education, there is a greater likelihood that if their children are in school their tenure will be short-lived and they are likely to begin work at an early age. This is especially true if children do not show academic promise. An underlying factor that influences this problem is expendable family resources. Children from poor families are often required to participate in accumulating resources for the family at an earlier age. The more time they have to spend contributing to the family's resource pool, the less time they have for school [68, 69].

Conclusions

As noted in ILO Convention 182, 'detailed information and statistical data on the nature and extent of child labour should be compiled and kept up to date to serve as a basis for determining priorities for national action for the abolition of child labour, in particular for the prohibition and elimination of its worst forms, as a matter of urgency' [20].

While studies on the health effects of child labour may be lacking, compelling data describe the potential harmful effects of contaminants on children and their communities. However, even well-designed studies may not readily distinguish between harm resulting directly from work and harm resulting from social inequalities or the ambient environment. This will remain a challenge into the foreseeable future.

In order to gain a better understanding of the impact of child labour on health, there is a need for more and better-designed studies and surveillance systems. Studies should include appropriate sample sizes, comparison groups, and clear definitions of hazardous exposures and outcomes. Such studies are hard to design, and many hazards are difficult and expensive to measure. Given the difficulties and cost in carrying out studies, it is important to more effectively use existing epidemiological and occupational health data in defining and identifying harmful work. In addition, it is important to conduct ongoing surveillance programmes to determine the nature and prevalence of work-related injuries and illnesses.

Harmful work affects individual children and adolescents through a loss of opportunity (e.g. education) and the development of premature illness and disability. Industrial and agricultural processes have significant potential to erode the quality of life for all community members. The examination of work processes should not neglect the possibility that both children and adults in surrounding communities may suffer from environmental contamination.

Public health workers and others may need to determine if children are being harmed by work, or if there is evidence that they are likely to be harmed by work. This chapter provides a framework for understanding how work affects health and development in the individual as well as the community. It also provides a framework for understanding the long- and short-term consequences of different types of hazards.

Subsequent chapters present a detailed analysis of several types of problems and exposures. These include work-related injuries, lead exposure, silicosis and silico-tuberculosis, HIV/AIDS, and pesticide exposure. Together, these provide detailed examples of developmental problems, community health effects, as well as other acute and chronic health outcomes.

References

1 Graitcer PI, Lerer LB (1998). Child labor and health: quantifying the global health impacts of child labor. Washington, DC: The World Bank.

2 International Labour Office I. Forced labour. Available at http://www.ilo.org/global/Themes/Forced_Labour/lang–en/index.htm (accessed 2 September 2009).

3 Costa G (2005). [Health inequalities among occupations: epidemiologic hints for labour and social protection policies]. *La Medicina del lavoro*, **96**(Suppl):s7–27.

4 Hesketh T, Gamlin J, Woodhead M (2006). Policy in child labour. *Archives of disease in childhood*, **91**(9):721–3.

5 Goe SK, Henneberger PK, Reilly MJ, Rosenman KD, Schill DP, Valiante D, *et al.* (2004). A descriptive study of work aggravated asthma. *Occupational and Environmental Medicine*, **61**(6):512–7.

6 Henneberger PK, Hoffman CD, Magid DJ, Lyons EE (2002). Work-related exacerbation of asthma. *International Journal of Occupational and Environmental Health*, **8**(4):291–6.

7 Andersen SL (2003). Trajectories of brain development: point of vulnerability or window of opportunity? *Neuroscience and Biobehavioral Reviews*, **27**(1–2):3–18.

8 Rice DC (1998). Developmental lead exposure: neurobehavioral consequences. In Slikker W, Change LW (eds), *Handbook of Developmental Neurotoxicology*. New York: Academic Press.

9 Boyden J (1997). Constructing and reconstructing childhood. In James A, Prout A (eds), *Childhood and the Policy Makers, a Comparative Perspective on the Globalization of Childhood*, 2nd ed. London: Routledge Falmer.

10 Chang L, Guo G (1998). Fetal Minimata disease: Congenital methylmercury poisoning. In Slikker W, Chang LW (eds), *Handbook of Environmental Neurotoxicology*. New York: Academic Press.

11 Desaiah D (1998). Developmental toxicity of pesticides. In Slikker W, Chang LW (eds), *Handbook of Environmental Neurotoxicology*. New York: Academic Press.

12 Kassouf AL, McKee M, Mossialos E (2001). Early entrance to the job market and its effect on adult health: Evidence from Brazil. *Health Policy Plan*, **16**(1):21–8.

13 Laraqui CH, Caubet A, Laraqui O, Belamallem I, Harourate K, Curtes JP, *et al.* (2000). Child labor in the artisan sector of Morocco: Determinants and health effects. *Sante Publique*, 12(1):31–43.

14 Saddik B, Williamson A, Nuwayhid I, Black D (2005). The effects of solvent exposure on memory and motor dexterity in working children. *Public Health Reports*, **120**(6):657–63.

15 Teixeira LR, Fischer FM, Lowden A (2006). Sleep deprivation of working adolescents: A hidden work hazard. *Scandinavian Journal of Work, Environment & Health*, **32**(4):328–30.

16 Curcio G, Ferrara M, De Gennaro L (2006). Sleep loss, learning capacity and academic performance. *Sleep Medicine Reviews*, **10**(5):323–37.

17 Wigle D (2003). *Child health and the environment*. New York: Oxford University Press.

18 Schei MA, Hessen JO, Smith KR, Bruce N, McCracken J, Lopez V (2004). Childhood asthma and indoor woodsmoke from cooking in Guatemala. *Journal of Exposure Analysis and Environmental Epidemiology*, **14**(Suppl 1):S110–7.

19 Chen BH, Hong CJ, Pandey MR, Smith KR (1990). Indoor air pollution in developing countries. *World Health Statistics Quarterly*, **43**(3):127–38.

20 Gern JE, Rosenthal LA, Sorkness RL, Lemanske RF, Jr (2005). Effects of viral respiratory infections on lung development and childhood asthma. *The Journal of Allergy and Clinical Immunology*, **115**(4):668–74; quiz 75.

21 Sreedharan R, Mehta DI (2004). Gastrointestinal tract. *Pediatrics*, **113**(4 Suppl): 1044–50.

22 Weiss B (2006). Methylmercury: A model neurotoxicant and risk assessment dilemma. In Bellinger DC(ed.) *Human Developmental Neurotoxicology*. New York: Taylor & Francis.

23 Amler R, Smith L (2001). Achievements in children's environmental health. Atlanta, GA: US Department of Health and Human Services, Agency for Toxic Substances and Disease Registry.

24 Climatic heat stress and the exercising child and adolescent American Academy of Pediatrics. (2000). Committee on Sports Medicine and Fitness. *Pediatrics*, **106**(1 Pt 1): 158–9.

25 Levy BS, Wegman DH (2000). *Occupational health: Recognizing and prevention work-related disease and injury*. Philadelphia: Lippincott Williams and Wilkins.

26 Stellman JM (1998). Encyclopedia of Occupational Health and Safety, 4th ed. Geneva: International Labour Office.

27 Greenberg M (2003). *Occupational, industrial, and environmental toxicology*. Philadelphia: Mosby.

28 Forastieri V (1997). *Children at work: Health and safety risks*. Geneva: International Labour Office.

29 Weinberg JL, Bunin LJ, Das R (2009). Application of the industrial hygiene hierarchy of controls to prioritize and promote safer methods of pest control: a case study. *Public Health Reports*, **124**(Suppl 1):53–62.

30 Davidson PW, Myers GJ, Cox C, Axtell C, Shamlaye C, Sloane-Reeves J, *et al.* (1998). Effects of Prenatal and Postnatal Methylmercury Exposure From Fish Consumption on Neurodevelopment: Outcomes at 66 months of age in the Seychelles Child Development Study. *Journal of the American Medical Association*, **280**(8):701–7.

31 Kumar B, Gurung YB, Adhikari KP, Subedi G (2001). Nepal – situation of child ragpickers: A rapid assessment. Geneva: ILO.

32 Porto MF, Junca DC, Goncalves Rde S, Filhote MI (2004). [Garbage, work, and health: a case study of garbage pickers at the metropolitan landfill in Rio de Janeiro, Brazil]. Cadernos de saude publica / Ministerio da Saude, Fundacao Oswaldo Cruz, *Escola Nacional de Saude Publica*, **20**(6):1503–14.

33 Chien VC, Chai SK, Hai DN, Takaro T, Checkoway H, Keifer M, *et4294967295al.* (2002). Pneumoconiosis among workers in a Vietnamese refractory brick facility. *American Journal of Industrial Medicine*, **42**(5):397–402.

34 Rushton L (2007). Chronic obstructive pulmonary disease and occupational exposure to silica. *Reviews on Environmental Health*, **22**(4):255–72.

35 Li J, Shang X, Zhao Z, Tanguay RL, Dong Q, Huang C (2009). Polycyclic aromatic hydrocarbons in water, sediment, soil, and plants of the Aojiang River waterway in Wenzhou, China. *Journal of Hazardous Materials*, **173**(1–3):75–81.

36 Tariq SR, Shah MH, Shaheen N (2009). Comparative statistical analysis of chrome and vegetable tanning effluents and their effects on related soil. *Journal of hazardous materials*, **169**(1-3):285–90.

37 Perone A, Gelosa L (1982). [Findings on the spread of anthrax spores in the provincial territory of Milan with tanneries]. *Giornale di batteriologia, virologia ed immunologia*, **75**(7–12):322–36.

38 Ameen M, Musthapa S, Ahmad I, Ansari FA, Baig MA, Rahman Q (2003). Alteration in cellular and biochemical markers of pulmonary toxicity in rat lung exposed to carpet dusts. *Inhalation Toxicology*, 15(11):1119–31.

39 Green DA (2003). Lung function changes in teenage carpet weavers. *Indian Pediatrics*, **40**(3):221–5.

40 Choobineh A, Lahmi M, Shahnavaz H, Jazani RK, Hosseini M (2004). Musculoskeletal symptoms as related to ergonomic factors in Iranian hand-woven carpet industry and general guidelines for workstation design. *International Journal of Occupational Safety and Ergonomics*, **10**(2):157–68.

41 Joshi SK, Sharma U, Sharma P, Pathak SS, Sitaraman S, Verma CR (1994). Health status of carpet weaving children. *Indian Pediatrics*, **31**(5):571–4.

42 Mitra AK, Haque A, Islam M, Bashar SA (2009). Lead poisoning: an alarming public health problem in Bangladesh. *International Journal of Environmental Research and Public Health*, **6**(1):84–95.

43 Arcury TA, Vallejos QM, Schulz MR, Feldman SR, Fleischer AB, Jr., Verma A, *et al.* (2008). Green tobacco sickness and skin integrity among migrant Latino farmworkers. *American Journal of Industrial Medicine*, **51**(3):195–203.

44 Khan DA, Shabbir S, Majid M, Naqvi TA, Khan FA (2009). Risk assessment of pesticide exposure on health of Pakistani tobacco farmers. *Journal of Exposure Science & Environmental Epidemiology*, **20**(2):196–204.

45 National Research Council Institute of Medicine (1998). Protecting youth at work: Health, safety, and development of working children and adolescents in the United States. Washington DC: National Academy Press.

46 Janicak CA (1999). An analysis of occupational homicides involving workers 19 years old and younger. *Journal of Occupational and Environmental Medicine / American College of Occupational and Environmental Medicine*, **41**(12):1140–5.

47 Runyan CW, Bowling JM, Schulman M, Gallagher SS (2005). Potential for violence against teenage retail workers in the United States. *Journal of Adolescent Health*, **36**(3):267 e1–5.

48 Windau J, Sygnatur E, Toscano G (1999). Profile of work injuries incurred by young workers. *Monthly Labour Review*, **122**(6):3–10.

49 U.S. Congress, Office of Technology Assessment (1985). Reproductive health hazards in the workplace. Washington, DC: US Government Printing Office OTA-BA-266.

50 Human Rights Watch (2000). Fingers to the Bone. Available at: http://www.hrw.org/en/reports/2000/06/02/fingers-bone.

51 National Institute for Occupational Safety and Health (NIOSH) (1997). Child labor research needs: Report of the Child Labor Research Group. Cincinnati, OH: NIOSH.

52 Barboza D (2003). Children scavenge a life, of sorts, in the garbage. *New York Times.* 25 August.

53 Parker DL, Carl WR, French LR, Martin FB (1994). Nature and incidence of self-reported adolescent work injury in Minnesota. *American Journal of Industrial Medicine*, **26**(4):529–41.

54 Mull LD, Kirkhorn SR (2005). Child labor in Ghana cocoa production: Focus upon agricultural tasks, ergonomic exposures, and associated injuries and illnesses. *Public Health Reports*, **120**(6):649–55.

55 McKnight RH, Spiller HA (2005). Green tobacco sickness in children and adolescents. *Public Health Reports* **120**(6):602–5.

56 Faden R (1985). Reproductive health hazards in the workplace. Washington D.C.: Office of Technology Assessment.

57 Gunn S, Zenaida O (1992). Dilemmas in tackling child labour: The case of scavenger children in the Philippines. *International Labor Review*, **131**(6):629–46.

58 Sinha S (1991). *Child Labour in Calcutta: A sociological study*. Calcutta: Naya Prokash.

59 O'Leary D (1998). *A Socioeconomic Study of Waste Pickers in Phnom Penh* [monograph]. Phnom Penh: The Community Sanitation & Recycling Organization, Centre for Social Development.

60 Nuwayhid IA, Usta J, Makarem M, Khudr A, El-Zein A (2005). Health of children working in small urban industrial shops. *Occupational and Environmental Medicine*, **62**(2):86–94.

61 Human Rights Watch (2002). Child labor in Agriculture. New York [updated 2002; cited 2009 August 30]; Availableat http://www.hrw.org/en/reports/2002/06/11/child-labor-agriculture.

62 Mkandawire-Valhmu L, Rodriguez R, Ammar N, Nemoto K (2009). Surviving life as a woman: A critical ethnography of violence in the lives of female domestic workers in Malawi. *Health Care for Women International*, **30**(9):783–801.

63 Cheng SJ (1996). Migrant women domestic workers in Hong Kong, Singapore and Taiwan: a comparative analysis. *Asian and Pacific Migrations Journal*, **5**(1):139–52.

64 Weisssbrodt D (2008). *The Human Rights of Non-citizens.* New York: Oxford University Press.

65 Rama A, Rokade MA, Zingde D, Boroleb DV (2009). Post-depositional memory record of mercury in sediment near the effluent disposal site of a chlor-alkali plant in Thane Creek-Mumbai Harbour, India. *Environmental Technology*, **30**(8):765–83.

66 Sousa RN, Veiga MM (2009). Using performance indicators to evaluate an environmental education program in artisanal gold mining communities in the Brazilian Amazon. *Ambio*, **38**(1):40–6.

67 Bruce N, Perez-Padilla R, Albalak R (2000). Indoor air pollution in developing countries: A major environmental and public health challenge. *Bulletin of the World Health Organization*, **78**(9):1078–92.

68 Wolff FC, Maliki (2008). Evidence on the impact of child labor on child health in Indonesia, 1993–2000. *Economics and Human Biology*, **6**(1):143–69.

69 Post D, Pong S (2009). Student labour and academic proficiency in international perspective. *International Labour Review*, **148**(1–2):93–122.

Chapter 9A

Illustrative example A: Work-related injuries

Anaclaudia G. Fassa

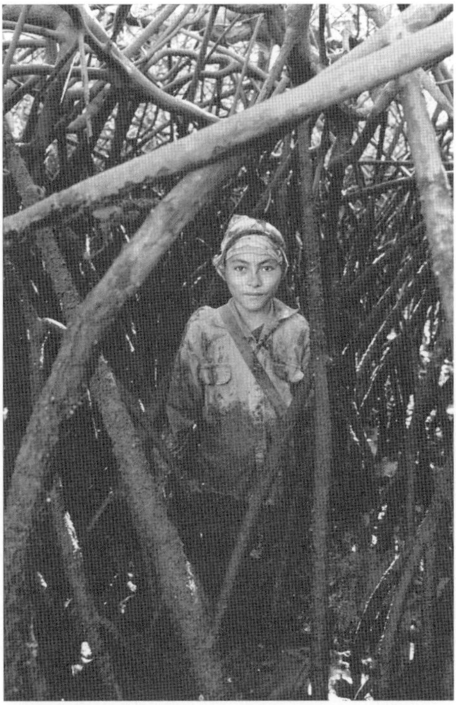

Conch shell digger, Nicaragua

Introduction

Many child and adolescent workers are injured at work. They suffer acute injuries with or without chronic consequences and sometimes injuries are fatal. In addition to their physical and psychological impacts, serious injuries have considerable financial and social impact which are even greater when the affected subjects are young. Work-related injuries in children and young workers therefore constitute an important public health concern. This chapter examines the frequency of work-related injuries in children and adolescents, their determinants and consequences, and the interventions that might address the problem.

Most of the available literature on child labour and injuries comes from developed countries, mainly from the United States and Canada. Even in developed countries, however, studies are limited. The majority of data is derived from the workers' compensation claims (WCC) databank which is limited to formal employees, aged over 15 years, who have suffered injuries that resulted in work leave. Eligibility requirements for WCC vary by state, particularly regarding duration of absence from work and severity of injury. This makes it difficult to compare studies. Identifying a denominator for injury events is problematic because of the part-time or seasonal nature of children and young people's work. Even in developed countries, data on informal workers, workers younger than 15 years old and the long-term effects of work-related injuries are limited [1, 2].

In developing countries, the quality of data is poorer still. Work-related injuries in formal employees are highly under-reported, and the number of informal workers is huge, particularly in agriculture where most child workers are found. Thus, the majority of studies in developing countries are descriptive surveys.

The magnitude of the problem

In the United States, approximately 230,000 young workers suffer a work-related injury each year and 77,000 require treatment in emergency departments [1]. In North America, the non-fatal injury rate in 14–17 year olds has been reported at around 5 per 100 full-time equivalent (FTE) workers [2, 3], but reaches 14 per 100 FTE in New Zealand [4]. By occupation, the non-fatal injury rate per 100 FTE workers (14–17 years) has been reported at: 6 for retail; 5 for manufacturing and construction; and 4 for agriculture and services [2], while for mining the male rate is estimated at 8 per 100 FTE workers respectively [5]. Among the few studies on workers younger than 14 years, work-related injury rates requiring medical attention or affecting daily activities varies from 2 to 6% [6, 7]. The prevalence of injuries is particularly high among children working on family farms or business (37% and 21% respectively), newspaper jobs (24%) and among those working for an individual doing services in the home (14%) [6].

In United States, on average 70 children die each year from work-related injuries and 30% of these occur in a family business, primarily farms. Agriculture accounts for 41% of US fatal work-related injuries to young people, followed by construction with 18% and retail and services with 13% each. In agriculture, two thirds of the fatalities resulted from transportation incidents; in retail settings about half are attributable to homicide; and in construction, falls and transportation incidents together account for two-thirds of the fatalities [8].

With regard to economically less-developed countries, a study from Brazil reported an annual incidence of work-related injuries of 8.5% for 10- to 17-year-old workers [9]. In the Philippines, the annual incidence has been estimated at 24% in 5- to 17-year-old, being higher for agricultural activities than for non-agricultural activities (32% and 14% respectively) [10].

The global burden of work-related injuries among young workers has been estimated in disability adjusted life years (DALYs). These estimates were based upon developed countries fatal and non-fatal injury rates by occupation and nature of injury. Working conditions in developing countries, however, are usually worse than in developed countries. Therefore, the reported figures may represent an under-estimate of the true overall figures. Each year, 2.7 million years of life are lost or lived with disability as a result of fatal and non-fatal work injuries in 5- to 17-year-olds; 70% of this DALYs occur in 5- to 14-years-old. Mining has the highest DALY rate (2.6 DALY per 100 FTE workers per year) followed by agriculture and construction (1.5 DALY per 100 FTE workers per year). However, reflecting working patterns, in terms of absolute numbers, agriculture has the highest number of years of life lost or lived with disability (1.91 million DALYs per year) [11].

The determinants of work-related injuries in young workers

The literature suggests an inverse association between work-related injuries and both age and socioeconomic status. There are also higher risks of injuries among males, migrants, and ethnic minority workers. One of the current challenges is to determine to what degree these associations are a result of occupational factors, and to what degree other factors are implicated in work-related injuries [12–14]. It is important also to consider the fact that adolescents are in a stage of development when some hazards might be potentiated (e.g. rapid growth and physical hazards, and higher sleep requirements and long hours of work or combining work and school) [12].

Age and gender

The majority of studies show that young workers have a higher non-fatal injury rate but a lower fatality rate than older workers [13, 15]. These associations vary by gender with young men having a consistently higher injury rate than older men; whereas for women the results are inconsistent [15]. Young injured workers have proportionally more acute traumatic injuries and fewer musculoskeletal injuries than older workers [13]. The age-related differences are reduced when job characteristics such as type of occupation and level of physical exertion required are controlled for, but a moderately elevated risk persists. This residual risk might be explained by other occupational hazards, such as differences in workplace environment or organizational structure as well as physical and cognitive developmental factors [13].

Studies consistently show that the adolescent injury rate for males is nearly double that for females (7 and 4.4 per 100 FTE workers respectively) [2, 12]. However, industry-specific studies (e.g. retail) show no gender differences in youth injury rates suggesting that reported gender differences rates are strongly associated with the type of work [16]. Most studies that control the association for job and workplace factors do not present a gender independent association with work-related injuries [17].

Education

There is consistent evidence of the association between low educational status and work-related injuries. The prevalence of work-related injuries among young workers is 30% higher when their mothers have the lowest level of education when compared to those with the highest level of education. Moreover, adolescents who work to support their families have demonstrated 25% more work-related injuries than those that do not support their families [18]. Young people who are out of school show a 1.5- to 3-fold increased risk of work-related injuries, compared to students. Moreover, education level is inversely associated with work-related injury rates. These associations persist after adjustment for demographic and work factors [14, 19]. Job characteristics, such as increased physical exertion and working in sales and service or manual occupations, partly explain this gradient in education, but there is a residual risk that might be related to work aspects not considered in the studies, or factors other than education per se [14, 19, 20]. However, education might have also a direct effect in work injury risks. The causal mechanism is not fully understood.

Migrant workers and ethnic minority groups

Migrant students are 2 to 4 times more likely to report a work-related injury when compared to working students from families that did not migrate [21]. Ethnic minority young workers (Hispanic and African-American) have 67 to 80% more work-related injuries than their white peers [6, 22]. The risk of severe injuries in ethnic minority teenage workers has ranged from 1.6 to 3 times the risk in white working teenagers [22, 23]. Moreover, inadequate access to health services might worsen the consequences of a work-related injury. In contrast, a Canadian study reported that white respondents were 59% more likely to sustain a work-related injury than ethnic minorities (Black, Asian, and Aboriginal) [14]. The effects might vary because ethnic minorities are a heterogeneous group. For example, among Hispanics, US-raised bilingual adolescents might have a lower risk of injury than recent immigrants [24].

The factors that mediate the association between ethnic minority/migrant worker status and work-related injuries are not fully determined. In similar occupations, Hispanic and African-American teenagers were more likely to report working more than 23 hours per week and to work past 11:00 pm when compared with white teenagers [22]. Moreover, US Hispanics have a much higher school drop-out rate than other ethnic groups and only 57% of Hispanics (age 25 years and over) have completed high school (US Census). Thus, it is likely that there is a complex interaction between educational and economic disadvantages, cultural barriers such as language which limits training and supervision, as well as differences in occupational hazards exposure even when in similar occupations.

Occupational factors

Several descriptive studies show that young workers are exposed to multiple occupational hazards. Surprisingly, considering the range of hazards, few analytical studies have examined the association between occupational hazards and work-related injury in young people [17, 25]. Work setting serves as a proxy for the composite of hazards that exists in the workplace [26].

When compared to young people employed in administrative and clerical jobs, those working in sales and service jobs, trade/transport, farming/forestry / fishing, and process/manufacturing occupations are 2 to 4 times more likely to be injured at work [14, 20].

In Brazil, young people working in manufacturing and domestic services had a higher risk of musculoskeletal pain and back pain than those not working. These adverse outcomes were a result of awkward postures as well as monotonous or heavy physical work [27]. A cold or dangerous workplace, toxic exposures, increased physical exertion, and psychological job demands have all been associated with work-related injuries in young people [20, 28]. In the Philippines, short-term workers have demonstrated an increased risk of non-fatal injury when compared to permanent workers; while in agricultural activities, seasonal workers also present a high risk [10].

About half of adolescents injured at work in the USA have received no safety training [29]. Some studies have found that longer working hours and working after 11:00 pm increases the likelihood of a work-related injury [14, 23, 30], while others have not found this association [17]. Being rushed at work has also been found to increase the risk of injury in young people [26].

A higher risk of work-related injuries might be anticipated in the informal market. In Brazil, 85% of 10–17 year old workers are informal workers [27, 31]. In the United States, 30% of the young people do not have work permits. However, teenagers with work permits have been no less likely to be injured than those without permits and no less likely to have a near-miss incident [31]. Despite the fact that teenagers with work permits are more likely to be given safety training, more than 35% of the young workers perform tasks prohibited for persons of their age [25, 32].

In US agriculture, where family farms are exempt from regulations, 24% of injuries involve family children and of those injured children, more than 30% have been performing work prohibited under the hazardous occupations orders [33]. Law enforcement and better monitoring of family work might help reduce work-related injuries among young workers.

Risk markers

Young people that have experienced a 'near-miss' incident at work, are 6 times more likely to experience a work-related injury than their peers. Having a co-worker injured and being asked to do something dangerous, more than doubles the risk of work-related injury [6, 30]. These variables seem to be important risk markers for work injury and could be used to prevent future incidents.

Risk perception

Adolescents

Minor, frequent, low severity injuries may be seen as 'part of the job' [16]. Traditionally, studies have attributed the risks taken by teenagers to their perceptions of invulnerability and lack of ability to assess hazards. However, recent studies show that young people and adults share a similar optimism about their ability to avoid harm and learn from experience at the same pace. Young workers recognize the hazards at the workplace, but compared to adult workers, they tend to underestimate the risks associated with them [3, 13, 16, 24].

This underestimation of risk may also reflect young workers' powerlessness. Studies suggest that teenagers are too intimidated to voice their concerns to managers; they feel vulnerable, afraid of being fired, and they have the perception that managers lack concern about workplace safety [34]. It has also been found that female workers' concerns are dismissed by managers, and complaints about female jobs are delegitimized by managers who suggest that these jobs are less demanding than male jobs. On the other hand, young male workers do not complain or report injuries, and neglect to ask for help. Males adopt these strategies to prove themselves as mature, capable workers [16].

These findings suggest that programmes focusing exclusively on educating young workers about their rights will have a limited effect on safety at work. In order to improve occupational safety, it is important to consider wider gender and power relationships, as well as the key role of managers [16].

Parents

In a study of US parents, 90% agreed that young workers learn valuable job skills and are less likely to get into trouble than teenagers who don't work [35]. On family farms, parents believe that the work brings about a sense of responsibility and self-confidence, teaches useful knowledge, skills, cooperation, and teamwork, and brings families closer together [36].

Between 30 and 50% of the parents expressed concern about young workers being at work during a robbery, not receiving safety training, working alone, not getting enough sleep, getting physically or sexually assaulted, working too late at night, not using protective equipment, being rushed at work, doing hazardous tasks, or handling hazardous equipment or substances. However, just 13% were concerned that working could be dangerous for their teenage child [35]. Among farm parents who considered farming more dangerous than other occupations, 25% did not consider children working on a farm more dangerous when compared to other work in which they might be engaged. Thus, for parents, the benefits outweigh the risks and while they perceive some occupations as dangerous, they rationalize hazards and do not take safety actions nor advise that their teenagers do the same [36].

Almost all parents thought that the law should limit equipment use and the kinds of tasks teenagers are allowed to do. Approximately 85% thought teenagers should work 20 hours or less a week, but 35% felt that 16–17 year olds could work after 10 pm [35]. Another study explored parental beliefs about the importance of considering developmental characteristics when evaluating children's readiness to perform new tasks. Parental safety beliefs were not associated with such task assignment. However, the belief in the importance of 'physical readiness' (age and size) reduced agricultural injury risk in 20% while the belief in the importance of 'cognitive readiness' (maturity and skills) reduced the injury risk in 70% for females but was not associated with males' risk [37].

Parents do recognize safety and health problems in their children's work. However, there is an important disconnection between this knowledge and any safety actions. This also has implications for improving parents' ability to advise their children on safety and health issues and in the selection of age-appropriate jobs.

The long-term impact of work-related injuries

Health

Few studies have evaluated the long-term health impact of work-related injuries in children and young people. In the United States, the prevalence of injuries resulting in two or more missed working days varied from 15 to 47% in studies of workers' compensation claims [29, 38-42], and 26% of young workers reported ongoing medical problems. Permanent impairment such as chronic pain, scarring, sensory loss, and loss of range of motion occurred in 15–44% of injured young people [40, 41, 43]. Both males and females demonstrated an increase in health care use immediately after a work-related injury. For males, after adjusting for age, occupation, socioeconomic status, and geographic location, musculoskeletal injuries increased the chance of requiring health care [44].

Economic consequences

As well as their immediate effects on individuals and families, work-related injuries have important wider social and economic costs. In 1993 in the United States, the direct (e.g. medical costs, workplace disruption) and indirect (e.g. lifetime earnings losses) occupational injuries costs were estimated at US $5 billion: approximately 3% of the total of injury costs involving teenagers [45]. A Canadian case–control study, matched on the basis of earnings, showed that young workers experiencing a work-related disability, which required an absence of 5 working days or more, had significantly fewer earnings than the controls in the year after the absence. This association was not due to between-group differences in school activity or working hours. The mean difference in earnings, in the year following the absence, between the cases and controls was CAD $1015 (US $938). This means that injured workers earned 6.7% less than the controls. It is not clear to what extent these losses were related to residual work disability, injury-related job loss, or the stigma attached to work disability, or for how long such earnings losses persist [46].

Interventions to reduce work-related injuries

Education and training, enforcement of relevant occupational health and safety regulation, and engineering out hazards where possible are important injury prevention strategies [19].

Education and training

Canada and the United States have invested in young workers' safety-training, but the coverage is low. Those that received training were no less likely to be injured than untrained working peers [24]. Recommended strategies to expand safety training include the incorporation of general safety education and training into the school curriculum [6]. However, since a substantial proportion of young people drop out before completing high school (25% in British Columbia), provision of information through media other than school must be considered. This could include workplace training/supervision and community-based social marketing programmes for vulnerable subgroups [19, 47].

To be more effective, safety training needs to be age and culturally appropriate [24]. Safety materials should focus on the main hazards. Moreover, since 10% of injuries to young workers occur in the first week of employment, and a further 10% occur in the subsequent 3 weeks it is important to provide training before young people start working [47]. Training should cover occupational health and safety subjects, as well as young workers' rights. It should also discuss how to deal with power relationships at work. Given the central role of managers and supervisors, it is important to provide them with occupational health and safety training emphasizing the importance of balanced power relationships in the prevention of injuries [16].

Regulation enforcement

Businesses that employ young workers assume a higher level of social obligation [12]. Thus, regulatory efforts should focus on the role of management in eliminating unsafe working conditions and ensuring the protection of young workers [16]. Moreover, near-miss incidents at work or an injury in any co-worker should be considered as a serious untoward incident and trigger further preventive actions [30].

Enforcement of occupational health and safety regulation, such as prohibiting teenagers from working long and late hours during the school week may be one method to reduce severe injuries in young people [30]. Legislation enforcement must be associated with education to avoid migration of workers to informal, more hidden, unsafe occupations. Where constraints are placed on employment opportunities, particularly in developed countries, young people might spend more time in recreational activities, some of which may be more likely to result in injury. Risk trade-offs must be taken into consideration and policies that enhance the safety of recreational activities might be important to reduce the total injury burden across this age group [48].

Cultural attitudes

There is currently debate about the need to expand regulations to family work, mainly to those on family farms [36]. If legislative enforcement is already difficult in situations of employment, it will be more difficult within a family. Efforts to address attitudes and change behaviour may be a better approach to this problem. These efforts should comprise a two-way dialogue, so that solutions are appropriate for each situation and acquired knowledge results in sustained family's engagement on occupational health and safety.

Eliminating job hazards

A substantial portion of young people's injury risk appears to be modifiable through addressing job hazards. The elimination or control of hazards through engineering, appropriate supervision, and training are very important strategies, however, they are often underused[13]. The elimination or control of hazards is particularly important strategy because it has a permanent effect, benefiting all workers and raising standards regarding what is acceptable at work.

Conclusions

Work-related injuries in young people comprise an important public health problem that results in a considerable social, economic, and health burden for individuals and society. Males, migrants, ethnic minority workers, younger workers, and those with lower education levels present a higher risk of work-related injuries. This association is mediated, at least in part, by occupation and hazards. Agriculture is the most common form of work among children, carrying a high risk of injuries and exposure to several important hazards.

Due to the scarcity of data from developed countries, it is necessary to evaluate to what extent findings from developing countries can be extrapolated to developing countries. Existing data suggest that work-related injury rates in young people are probably higher in developing countries. This reflects socio-demographic characteristics of workers, occupational profiles, and the prevalence of hazards. In many developing countries there is already a considerable amount of technology available, which combined with low education, poor training, and inadequate maintenance increases the risk of injuries. Moreover, poorer working conditions and higher physical requirements also increase the risk of injuries. Knowledge from developed countries about the determinants of work-related injuries in young people can therefore, to a considerable extent, be extrapolated to developing countries.

Descriptive studies and surveillance data are required in developing countries to examine and understand the specificities of injuries to children and young workers. This should include the evaluation of the prevalence of hazards and work-related injuries among young workers, as well as examining occupations that are not common in developed countries. Further studies are also necessary to better understand the complex set of determinants of young workers' injuries.

Interventions to prevent work injuries should include the 3E's (Education and training, Enforcement of occupational and safety regulations, and Engineering out the hazards) [19]. However, it is important to emphasize the responsibilities of managers and supervisors in preventing work-related injuries in young workers. As Holizki asserted in 2008, almost all serious injuries to young workers are preventable; it is an ethical imperative to prevent as many of these serious injuries as possible [47].

References

1 National Institute for Occupational Safety and Health (2003). NIOSH alert: Preventing deaths injuries and illnesses of young workers. Washington, DC: US Department of Health and Human Services.

2 Layne LA, Castillo DN, Stout N, Cutlip P (1994). Adolescent occupational injuries requiring hospital emergency department treatment: A nationally representative sample. *American Journal of Public Health*, **84**(4):657–60.

3 Chapeskie KFB (2003). Securing a safe and healthy future: The road to injury prevention for Ontario's young workers. *Institute for Work and Health (IWH), Infocus – Workplace Research Supplement* **34**:1–4.

4 Dufort VM, Kotch JB, Marshall SW, Waller AE, Langley JD (1997). Occupational injuries among adolescents in Dunedin, New Zealand, 1990–1993. *Annals of Emergency Medicine*, **30**(3):266–73.

5 Schober S, Handke J, Halperin W, Moll M, Thun M (1988). Work-related injuries in minors. *American Journal of Industrial Medicine*, **14**(5):585–95.

6 Zierold KM, Garman S, Anderson H (2004). Summer work and injury among middle school students, aged 10-14 years. *Occupational and Environmental Medicine*, **61**(6): 518–22.

7 Breslin FC, Koehoorn M, Cole DC (2008). Employment patterns and work injury experience among Canadian 12 to 14 year olds. *Canadian Journal of Public Health*, **99**(3):201–5.

8 Windau J, Mayer S (2005). Occupational injuries among young workers. *Monthly Labor Review*, **128**(10):11–23.

9 Santana V, Itaparica M, de Amorim AM, Araujo Filho JB, Araujo G, Oliveira M, *et al.* (2003). Non-fatal work-related accidents in adolescents. *Cademos de Saúde Pública*, **19**(2):407–20.

10 Castro CL, Gormly S, Ritualo AR (2005). The SIMPOC Philippine survey of children 2001: A data source for analyzing occupational injuries to children. *Public Health Reports*, **120**(6):631–40.

11 Fassa AG (2003). *Health Benefits of Eliminating Child Labour*. Geneva: ILO.

12 National Research Council-Institute of Medicine (1998). Protecting youth at work: Health, safety, and development of working children and adolescents in the United States. Washington DC: National Academy Press.

13 Breslin FC, Smith P (2005). Age-related differences in work injuries: A multivariate, population-based study. *American Journal of Industrial Medicine*, **48**(1):50–6.

14 Breslin FC, Smith P, Mustard C, Zhao R (2006). Young people and work injuries: An examination of jurisdictional variation within Canada. *Injury Prevention*, **12**(2): 105–10.

15 Salminen S (2004). Have young workers more injuries than older ones? An international literature review. *Journal of Safety Research*, **35**(5):513–21.

16 Breslin FC, Polzer J, MacEachen E, Morrongiello B, Shannon H (2007). Workplace injury or "part of the job"?: Towards a gendered understanding of injuries and complaints among young workers. *Social Science & Medicine*, **64**(4):782–93.

17 Breslin FC, Day D, Tompa E, Irvin E, Bhattacharyya S, Clarke J, *et al.* (2007). Non-agricultural work injuries among youth: A systematic review. *American Journal of Preventive Medicine*, **32**(2):151–62.

18 Rauscher KJ, Myers DJ (2008). Socioeconomic disparities in the prevalence of work-related injuries among adolescents in the United States. *Journal of Adolescent Health*, **42**(1):50–7.

19 Breslin FC (2008). Educational status and work injury among young people: Refining the targeting of prevention resources. *Canadian Journal of Public Health*, **99**(2):121–4.

20 Karmakar SD, Breslin FC (2008). The role of educational level and job characteristics on the health of young adults. *Social Science & Medicine*, **66**(9):2011–22.

21 Cooper SP, Weller NF, Fox EE, Cooper SR (2005). Comparative description of migrant farmworkers versus other students attending rural south Texas schools: substance use, work, and injuries. *Journal of Rural Health*, **21**(4):361–6.

22 Zierold S, Anderson HA (2006). Racial and ethnic disparities in work-related injuries among teenagers. *Journal of Adolescent Health*, **39**(3):422–6.

23 Weller NF, Cooper SP, Tortolero SR, Kelder SH, Hassan S (2003). Work-related injury among south Texas middle school students: prevalence and patterns. *Southern Medical Journal*, **96**(12):1213–20.

24 Young M, Rischitelli DG (2006). Occupational risks and risk perception among Hispanic adolescents. *McGill Journal of Medicine*, **9**(1):49–53.

25 Runyan CW, Dal Santo J, Schulman M, Lipscomb HJ, Harris TA (2006). Work hazards and workplace safety violations experienced by adolescent construction workers. *Archives of Pediatrics and Adolescent Medicine*, **160**(7):721–7.

26 Evensen CT, Schulman MD, Runyan CW, Zakocs RC, Dunn KA (2000). The downside of adolescent employment: Hazards and injuries among working teens in North Carolina. *Journal of Adolescence*, **23**(5):545–60.

27 Fassa AG, Facchini LA, Dall'Agnol MM, Christiani DC (2005). Child labor and musculoskeletal disorders: Pelotas, Brazil) epidemiological survey. *Public Health Reports*, **120**(6):665–73.

28 Fischer FM, Oliveira DC, Nagai R, Teixeira LR, Lombardi Junior M, Latorre MR, *et al* (2005). Job control, job demands, social support at work and health among adolescent workers. *Revista de Saude Publica*, **39**(2):245–53.

29 Knight E, Castillo D, Layne L (1995). A detailed analysis of work-related injury among youth treated in emergency departments. *American Journal of Industrial Medicine*, **27**(6):793–805.

30 Zierold KM, Anderson HA (2006). Severe injury and the need for improved safety training among working teens. *American Journal of Health Behavior*, **30**(5):525–32.

31 Zierold KM, Anderson H (2006). The relationship between work permits, injury, and safety training among working teenagers. *American Journal of Industrial Medicine*, **49**(5):360–6.

32 Rauscher KJ, Runyan CW, Schulman MD, Bowling JM (2008). US child labor violations in the retail and service industries: Findings from a national survey of working adolescents. *American Journal of Public Health*, **98**(9):1693–9.

33 Marlenga B, Berg RL, Linneman JG, Brison RJ, Pickett W (2007). Changing the child labor laws for agriculture: Impact on injury. *American Journal of Public Health*, **97**(2):276–82.

34 Zakocs RC, Runyan CW, Schulman MD, Dunn KA, Evensen CT (1998). Improving safety for teens working in the retail trade sector: Opportunities and obstacles. *American Journal of Industrial Medicine*, **34**(4):342–50.

35 Runyan CW, Schulman M, Dal Santo J, Bowling JM, Agans R (2009). Attitudes and beliefs about adolescent work and workplace safety among parents of working adolescents. *Journal of Adolescent Health*, **44**(4):349–55.

36 Zentner J, Berg RL, Pickett W, Marlenga B (2005). Do parents' perceptions of risks protect children engaged in farm work? *Preventive Medicine*, **40**(6):860–6.

37 Larson-Bright M, Gerberich SG, Masten AS, Alexander BH, Gurney JG, Church TR, *et al.* (2009). Parents' safety beliefs and childhood agricultural injury. *American Journal of Industrial Medicine*, **52**(9):724–33.

38 Miller ME, Kaufman JD (1998). Occupational injuries among adolescents in Washington State, 1988–1991. *American Journal of Industrial Medicine*, **34**(2):121–32.

39 Cooper SP, Burau KD, Robison TB, Richardson S, Schnitzer PG, Fraser JJ, Jr (1999). Adolescent occupational injuries: Texas, 1990–1996. *American Journal of Industrial Medicine*, **35**(1):43–50.

40 Parker DL, Carl WR, French LR, Martin FB (1994). Nature and incidence of self-reported adolescent work injury in Minnesota. *American Journal of Industrial Medicine*, **26**(4):529–41.

41 Parker DL, Carl WR, French LR, Martin FB (1994). Characteristics of adolescent work injuries reported to the Minnesota Department of Labor and Industry. *American Journal of Public Health*, **84**(4):606–11.

42 Runyan CW, Zakocs RC (2000). Epidemiology and prevention of injuries among adolescent workers in the United States. *Annual Review of Public Health*, **21**:247–69.

43 Belville R, Pollack SH, Godbold JH, Landrigan PJ (1993). Occupational injuries among working adolescents in New York State. *Journal of the American Medical Association*, **269**(21):2754–9.

44 Koehoorn M, Breslin FC, Xu F (2008). Investigating the longer-term health consequences of work-related injuries among youth. *Journal of Adolescent Health*, **43**(5):466–73.

45 Miller TRW, G. M (1998). Costs of occupational injuries to teenagers, United States. *Injury Prevention*, **4**(3):211–7.

46 Breslin FC, Tompa E, Zhao R, Amick BC, 3rd, Pole JD, Smith P, *et al.* (2007). Work disability absence among young workers with respect to earnings losses in the following year. *Scandinavian Journal of Work, Environment & Health*, **33**(3):192–7.

47 Holizki T, McDonald R, Foster V, Guzmicky M (2008). Causes of work-related injuries among young workers in British Columbia. *American Journal of Industrial Medicine*, **51**(5):357–63.

48 Breslin FC, Karmakar SD, Smith P, Etches J, Mustard C (2007). Time allocation between work and recreation and the associated injury risks among young people. *Journal of Safety Research*, **38**(3):373–9.

Chapter 9B

Illustrative example B: Pesticide exposure

Ana Maria Osorio

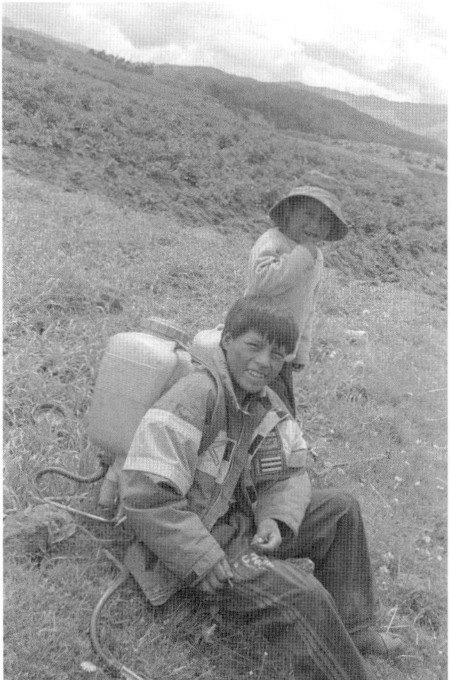

Pesticide sprayer, Peru

Introduction

It is estimated that 70% of child labourers (less than 18 years old) are employed in agriculture. These roughly 150 million children are more likely to be found in highly agricultural developing countries, especially in sub-Saharan Africa,

Asia, and the Pacific[1, 2]. Pesticide exposure is one of multiple hazards that young agricultural workers may face.

Table 9B.1 lists the percentage of the workforce in agriculture for selected countries. Developing countries such as Ethiopia, India, and Indonesia, can have some of the highest values and have a relatively younger population. In comparison, the US has 0.6% of the labour force employed in agriculture with a high median age of 36.7 years, and Argentina has 1.0% and 29.7 years, respectively [3]. In highly agricultural developing countries, having a relatively younger population may indicate a larger number of children working in the fields, accompanying their parents to work, and experiencing non-intentional bystander exposures when playing or living near areas where pesticides are applied. While there may be other routes of exposure leading to childhood pesticide intoxication, agriculture and the issue of child and adolescent farm workers play a major role in many developing countries.

These childhood pesticide intoxications are preventable. Since early manifestations are often not clinically recognized, it is very important to prevent exposure before significant and permanent health effects can develop. This chapter explores the relationship between children's health and pesticide exposure in developing countries, the different pesticide types and exposure, pesticide-associated health effects, intoxication case reports, preventive measures, and disease monitoring.

Table 9B.1 Percent of labour force in agriculture for selected countries [3]

	Population in 1000[a]	**Median age in years[b]**	**% Labour force in agriculture**	**Ref year estimate**
Argentina	40,482	29.7	1.0	2008
Belize	300	20.1	19.5	2005
Brazil	196,343	28.3	20.0	2003
Chile	16,454	31.1	13.2	2005
Costa Rica	4,196	27.1	14.0	2006
Egypt	81,714	24.5	32.0	2001
Ethiopia	82,545	16.9	80.2	2005
India	1,147,996	25.1	60.0	2003
Indonesia	237,512	27.2	42.1	2005
Mexico	109,955	26.0	15.1	2005
Philippines	96,062	22.3	35.0	2008
South Africa	48,783	24.2	9.0	2007
USA	303,825	36.7	0.6	2007

[a]2009 estimate

[b]2008 estimate.

Types of pesticides

The Food and Agriculture Organization (FAO) defines a pesticide as any substance or mixture of substances intended for preventing, destroying, repelling, or mitigating any pest [4]. These substances can be grouped according to the intended target pest or manner of delivery:

- *Fumigants* have a great capacity for diffusion onto target pest
- *Fungicides* work on mold and mildew
- *Herbicides* act as weed killers and defoliants
- *Insecticides* kill insects
- *Rodenticides* kill rats and other rodents
- *Wood treatment products* are used as wood preservatives

The World Health Organization (WHO) pesticide classification is based on acute animal toxicity studies using LD_{50} values. These values represent the number of mg of toxicant (pesticide) per kg of body weight needed to kill 50% of a large population of test animals, usually rats receiving oral dosing. The lower the LD_{50}, the more hazardous the substance [5]. There are four WHO classes:

- Ia – Extremely hazardous
- Ib – Highly hazardous
- II – Moderately hazardous
- III – Slightly hazardous

There are fumigants for which there is no classification because the WHO scheme applies only to oral and dermal exposure test dosing. Nonetheless, WHO recognizes fumigants such as methyl bromide as being a high level health hazard [5]. All other pesticides not classified are considered unlikely to be hazardous under normal use. Table 9B.2 lists a selection of pesticides with their respective WHO class designation. Within developing countries, the small scale farmers working in tropical climates will be more likely to use large amounts of the more toxic pesticides (WHO Class Ia, Ib, and II).

The persistent organic pollutants (POPs) are a pesticide group of special interest due to their tendency to remain in the environment for long periods of time, concentrate in fatty tissues, and bioaccumulate in food chains. Furthermore, children are at risk via breastfeeding and in utero exposures. Under the auspices of the UNEP (United Nations Environment Programme), there are international agreements for reducing and eliminating twelve POPs: aldrin, chlordane, dichlorodiphenyltrichloroethane (DDT), dieldrin, endrin, heptachlor, mirex, toxaphene, and hexachlorobenzene [6].

The Rotterdam Convention on Prior Informed Consent Procedure (PIC) for Certain Hazardous Chemicals and Pesticides in International Trade was

Table 9B.2 WHO pesticide classification examples [5]

Pesticide name	Type of pesticide	WHO class	LD_{50}
Aldicarb	Carbamate	Ia	0.93 mg/kg
Malathion	Insecticide	III	2100 mg/kg
Metam sodium	Fungicide	II	285 mg/kg
Methyl bromide	Fumigant	–[a]	–
Paraquat	Herbicide	II	50 mg/kg
Parathion	Insecticide	Ia	13 mg/kg
Pentachlorophenol	Wood treatment	Ib	80 mg/kg D[b]
Warfarin	Rodenticide	Ib	10 mg/kg

[a]fumigant recognized as a high hazard but non-classifiable per WHO scheme.
[b]D designates dermal route of dosing to obtain LD_{50}.

adopted in 1998. This convention gives importing countries the power to decide which potentially hazardous chemicals they want to receive and which they choose to exclude because they cannot manage them safely. As exemplified Table 9B.3, there are 39 chemicals covered by the convention and 28 of these are pesticides. These pesticides have been banned or severely restricted in many countries due to human health or environmental concerns. The higher risk pesticides are often exported from industrialized to developing nations [7].

Pesticide exposure

An individual may be exposed to pesticides via dermal contact (including ocular exposure), inhalation, ingestion, in utero contact, and breast feeding. Organophosphates, such as parathion, are examples of pesticides that can enter the body by all five of these exposure routes. Certain high risk scenarios may result in exposure for both adults and their children: small scale family farms, large commercial farms, bystander exposure via playing or living near fields being treated, farm workers taking hazardous farm chemicals home for private use, and farm workers bringing pesticide residues home on work clothes or shoes. Outside of agriculture, there may be leaks or spills from pesticide handling (production, storage, mixing, transport, or disposal activities), government-based vector control programmes, and inadequately trained pest control professionals [8].

The situation of young children and adolescents working as adults in agricultural fields deserves special mention. The farm setting may include the hazards of livestock handling, manure disposal, grain storage, heavy equipment use, and other hazardous tasks in addition to pesticide application and residue exposure. Hazardous pesticides may not be strictly controlled and

Table 9B.3 Pesticides listed in Rotterdam Convention [7]

2,4,5-T[a]	HCH[c]
Aldrin	Heptachlor
Binapacryl	Hexachlorobenzene
Captafol	Lindane
Chlordane	Mercury compounds[d]
Chlordimeform	Monocrotophos
Chlorobenzilate	Parathion
DDT	Pentachlorophenol[a]
Dieldrin	Toxaphene
Dinitro-ortho-cresol (DNOC)[b]	Dustable powder formulations containing benomyl, carbofuran, thiram[e]
Dinoseb[a]	Methamidophos[f]
1,2-dibromoethane (EDB)	Phosphamidon[g]
Ethylene dichloride	Methyl-parathion[h]
Ethylene oxide	
Fluoroacetamide	

[a]Includes salts and esters
[b]Includes salts such as ammonium salt, potassium salt and sodium salt
[c]Includes mixed isomers
[d]Includes inorganic mercury compounds, alkyl mercury compounds and alkyloxyalkyl and aryl mercury compounds
[e]Containing a combination of benomyl at or above 7%, carbofuran at or above 10%, thiram at or above 15%
[f]Soluble liquid formulations that exceed 600 g active ingredient/l
[g]Soluble liquid formulations that exceed 1000 g active ingredient/l, mixture of (E)&(Z) isomers, (Z)-isomer, and (E)-isomer
[h]Emulsifiable concentrates at or above 19.5% active ingredient and dusts at or above 1.5% active ingredient

there may be a lack of protective equipment when handling. The protective equipment, if available, may not fit correctly for adolescents. Studies in less industrialized countries indicate that farmers and presumably the youth working on the farms use very hazardous pesticides with usually no protective equipment [8, 17].

The special tasks that pose higher risks for adult workers also apply to youth doing adult work in the fields. For example, the leaking of pesticide onto clothing and skin during backpack spraying is associated with acute pesticide intoxication. Risk from this type of equipment is more likely when it doesn't fit the smaller frame of an adolescent, is not properly maintained, and the young person is not adequately trained. Additional risk factors often found in developing countries are the long work hours in hot and humid climates, possible mixing and loading of pesticide mixtures in delivery systems, or work in areas where pesticide have recently been applied. Finally, washing facilities or access to soap and water in agricultural settings is not often found. This results in day long exposure via contaminated clothing and skin, even while eating and drinking. The scenarios described are hazardous and associated with pesticide intoxication for children, adolescent, and adult farm workers [19].

Aside from the agricultural circumstances, there are other types of high-risk factors more frequently seen in developing countries: ability to purchase highly toxic pesticides intended for agricultural or professional pest control purposes on the open market or illegally (lack of regulation and enforcement), pesticide package instructions that are not in the local language or the pesticide is used in areas with a high degree of illiteracy, inability to afford personal protective equipment and clothing, and poor access to health care. Fatalities or near deaths from self-intoxication with pesticides are at higher levels in the developing world, and this event does occur among youths. In addition, highly toxic pesticides banned in the industrialized countries are coming into the developing world. However, there may be a lack of expertise or finances to properly store these highly toxic substances. Finally, many highly agricultural developing countries lack sufficient training about integrated pest management. This approach treats chemicals as only one part (and often the choice of last resort) of an overall plan to control pests. This training would be useful for persons participating in agricultural, commercial, domestic, and public health pest control activities [9]. By ensuring that pesticides are only used when needed, less toxic substances employed whenever possible and that all toxic material is handled appropriately, there will be less risk for exposing the most vulnerable part of the population, children, as well as adults.

Child health effects associated with pesticides

The human effects from pesticide exposure may be exacerbated when a child has concurrent health problems. For example, a child in a developing country may have intestinal parasites, suffer from malnutrition and dehydration, have latent TB, or be ill from other endemic illnesses. Poverty may play a role by putting the child into an unsafe and contaminated living situation and requiring the child to enter the workforce at a very young age. As noted elsewhere in this volume, there are some physiologic aspects that make children more vulnerable to pesticides or other environmental toxicants:

(1) Children breathe air, ingest food, and drink fluids at a higher per weight amount than adults. Thus, any pesticide contamination in the environment would result in a higher exposure for children than an adult.

(2) In the early years, children have metabolic systems that are less able to deal with toxicants like pesticides.

(3) There is multiple organ development in the prenatal period and childhood. These changing organ systems become more susceptible to environmental pesticide effects.

(4) Infants and young children are at an early developmental stage where objects are put into the mouth, and exploration of the environment may occur by crawling or walking into potentially contaminated surroundings [10, 11].

In industrialized nations with regional pesticide intoxication surveillance systems, the organophosphate insecticides tend to result in the most severe clinical presentations [12]. Although pesticide surveillance is not often found in highly agricultural developing countries, it is thought that organophosphates play a similar role in these nations.

The mechanism of action is the inhibition of the enzyme acetylcholinesterase (or cholinesterase) which breaks down the neurotransmitter acetylcholine. When this enzyme is inhibited, the acetylcholine is allowed to accumulate to excessively high levels. The range of problems associated with cholinesterase inhibition is seen in Table 9B.4. For children, the common presentation involves lethargy, coma, convulsions, flaccid muscle weakness, miosis, tachycardia, and excessive salivation. Pediatric patients present less often with bradycardia, fasciculations, lacrimation, and sweating as compared to adults [13, 14].

With respect to chronic disease conditions, there can be abnormal reproductive, child developmental, neurobehavioural, immunologic, endocrine disruption, and carcinogenic outcomes from different types of pesticides. The POP and PIC pesticides mentioned earlier have been associated with these abnormal conditions.

Table 9B.4 Possible health effects from cholinesterase inhibiting pesticides [13, 14]

	Physical signs and symptoms
Early onset	Headache, nausea, dizziness, lacrimation, sweating, salivation
More severe, later onset	Muscular twitch/fasciculations, weakness, tremor, incoordination, nausea, vomiting, abdominal cramps, diarrhoea
Ocular	Miosis (papillary constriction)
Neuropsychiatric	Anxiety, restlessness, depression, memory loss, confusion, psychosis
Respiratory	Bronchorrhea, bronchospasm, pulmonary oedema, respiratory depression and arrest (apnea)
Cardiovascular	Bradycardia and sinus arrest, tachycardia and hypertension, myocardiopathy
Advanced neurologic	Flaccid paralysis, loss of consciousness, incontinence, convulsions

Case reports

It is estimated that developing countries use a fourth of the world's production of pesticides, yet they experience 99% of the deaths [15]. However, there are very few pesticide intoxication monitoring programmes in place in developing countries and consequently little data in the literature about the extent of pesticide intoxications for most of the developing world.

The following are examples of estimated intoxication rates in developing countries: In 2006, Sri Lanka had a self-administration intoxication rate of approximately 180 cases per 100,000 and half of the 742 reported cases were associated with organophosphates. The case fatality rate was 10.9%. There was no detailed discussion of age among the study cases except to mention that adolescents were among the cases identified [16]. In 2002, the acute pesticide intoxication rate for Central America was estimated to be 15.8 cases per 100,000 inhabitants with a total of 712 fatalities. Table 9B.5 shows the unadjusted crude rate for reported acute pesticide intoxications for several Latin American countries. Caution should be used in comparing these results because there may have been variations in case definition and these are only crude rates. No information on age of the study group was provided [11].

Most incidence figures across countries are difficult to interpret because of different data collection methods and case ascertainment variability. To overcome these potential problems, PAHO coordinated a Central American project to assist each nation in establishing or enhancing existing regional

Table 9B.5 Examples of Pesticide Use and Reported Acute Pesticide Intoxications [11, 18] Figures represent the years 2000–2005

Country	Pesticide use in 1,000 kg[a]	Number of reported cases[b]	Population in 1,000[c]	Number of cases per 100,000 population[d]
Argentina	46,347	3,881	38,747	10.0
Bolivia	6,700	2,208	9,182	24.0
Brazil	131,970	4,273	186,831	2.3
Chile	24,197	804	44,946	6.1
Colombia	77,000	2,763	16,295	4.9
Ecuador	36,118	1,991	12,917	15.4
Uruguay	7,600	439	3,326	13.2

[a]Reference year is 2000 except for Argentina and Brazil (2002), and Ecuador (2004)
[b]Reference year is 2005 except for Bolivia (2000), Argentina and Brazil (2001), Uruguay (2002), and Ecuador (2004)
[c] Reference year is 2005
[d]Unadjusted crude rate

pesticide intoxication registries. The countries involved were Belize, Costa Rica, El Salvador, Guatemala, Honduras, Nicaragua, and Panama. This region represents 35 million inhabitants with 50% living in rural areas. For the age group less than 15 years old, there were 816 intoxication cases reported (5.7 per 100,000 population) with 27 fatalities (0.2 per 100,000 population) in the year 2000. This adolescent group had a smaller rate than the total population and there were a disproportionately higher number of males. Another aspect of this project was the analysis of under-reporting to each disease registry, e.g. number of cases not detected by the reporting system. The results for under-reporting of acute pesticide intoxications ranged from 77–99% of the true cases not detected [17].

In developing countries, children are frequently found working in agriculture. Surveillance data in Nicaragua indicated that 19% of acute occupational pesticide intoxication involved patients less than 16 years of age. It should be noted that 16 is the legal minimum age for working with pesticides in Nicaragua [20]. Another study in Nicaragua showed a higher pesticide intoxication rate for younger male workers and it was suggested that this was due to the lack of experience in this age group [21]. In a Costa Rican study, 5% of all intoxication cases on banana plantations were between 12 and 17 years of age [22]. However, even living in a farm household can be hazardous. In El Salvador, a study found an association between methyl parathion and acute symptoms (e.g. vomiting, dizziness, wheezing) in farmers who had recently applied the pesticide and family members who had not been involved in any field work [23].

Preventive measures and disease monitoring

Several steps may decrease the risk of childhood pesticide exposure. The main point to remember is that pesticide intoxication can be avoided so preventive measures should be emphasized in dealing with this public health problem. The following general recommendations may need to be adapted to address the specific national situations.

(1) Integrated pest management techniques should be adopted. Where possible, local residents, company owners, farmers, farm workers, and others who may be in contact with pesticides should be trained in this approach to pest management. The use of chemicals for pest control is a last resort.

(2) When used, the instruction for specific pesticides should be precisely followed. In cases of low literacy, or where instructions are not in the local language, farmers should be carefully instructed in their use.

(3) Public health and agricultural officials should work with their community leaders, school groups, and public health authorities to decrease and

eliminate potential pesticide exposures for children in all types of environments: home, school, work, and any other outside surroundings. Pediatric pesticide exposures should be prevented from occurring whenever possible.

(4) Pesticides and all dangerous products should be kept out of the reach of children at all times. Pesticides should be kept in secure and well-labeled containers, and, where possible, in locked cabinets.

(5) Families should be taught to use good hygienic practices when eating, storing, preparing and cooking food. Always wash food and your hands prior to ingestion, cooking and serving. Old containers should not be used for household chores.

(6) Public health and agricultural officials should question pest control professionals about safe work practices. Communities should mandate and enforce minimal application standards.

(7) In addition, community leaders, public health professionals and clinicians should address problems related to pesticide toxicity by taking the following steps:

  (1) Assist in reporting pesticide intoxication cases. If unfamiliar with the early signs and symptoms of an acute intoxication, obtain training and identify a specialist for future consultation, as needed.

  (2) Ensure that emergency care settings have clinicians skilled in dealing with pesticide intoxications, and adequate supplies of equipment, and medications

  (3) Distribute general information on pesticide intoxications to target high risk groups or geographic regions such as highly agricultural areas.

  (4) Work with policy makers to establish registration and control of pesticide sales and use if the country does not have these in place. In addition, consider the development of skilled professional pesticide applicators for commercial, agricultural, and public health pest control programmes. Development of a certificate programme for qualified pest control professionals should be considered.

  (5) Where possible, creating a monitoring programme for both pesticide use and sales, and pesticide-related illness would assist in tracking the extent of the problem and confirming that preventive measures are effective [8].

Conclusions

In the developing countries, the issue of children working in agriculture is common. For adult farm workers, the approach to preventing pesticide intoxication has included health and safety training, promotion of protective equipment, incorporation of integrated pest management, and training on safe handling of pesticides, when indicated. The prevention of farm-related child and adolescent occupational intoxications is even more problematic. The ideal solution would be to ban child farm workers and to enforce existing work age limits, where they exist. However, many factors contributing to the common occurrence of child farm labour in developing countries are difficult and often out of the control of the child worker. New approaches are needed to counter the higher rate of childhood pesticide intoxications in developing countries. One suggestion is to ban and enforce the most toxic pesticides and to promote and implement integrated pest management techniques [19]. One aspect is clear, this topic deserves a coordinated international effort from all sectors and from developed as well as developing countries.

Information resources

Pesticide classification and toxicology information

- International Program on Chemical Safety, WHO, ILO, and UNEP:
  http://www.who.int/ipcs/en
- Persistent Organic Pollutants (POPs), UNEP
  http://www.chem.unep.ch/pops/
- Prior Informed Consent (PIC) Procedure of the Rotterdam Convention, WHO, UNEP, and FAO:
  http://www.pic.int/home.php?type=t&id=5&sid=16

Diagnosis and treatment of pesticide intoxications

- EPA Recognition and Management of Pesticide Poisoning (in English and Spanish): www.epa.gov/pesticides/safety/healthcare/handbook/handbook.htm
- Case Studies in Environmental Medicine: Cholinesterase Inhibitors, ATSDR/CDC (online tutorial):www.atsdr.cdc.gov/csem/cholinesterase/contents.html

Pesticide-related disease monitoring

- INTOX program for poison centers and data collection: ww.who.int/ipcs/poisons/intox/en/index.html
- Proposed classification tool for acute pesticide intoxications, WHO www.who.int/bulletin/volumes/86/3/07-041814/en/

References

1 Hurst P (2007). Health and child labor in agriculture. *Food and Nutrition Bulletin*, **28**(Suppl 2):S364–71.

2 Hagemann F, Diallo Y, Etienne A, Mehran F (2006). *Global Child Labor Trends 2000 to 2004*, pp. 10, 17–18. Geneva: ILO.

3 CIA World Fact Report. Available at www.cia.gov/library/publications (accessed 5 Mar 2009).

4 FAO (2003). International code of conduct on the distribution and use of pesticides. FAO, Rome.

5 IPCS (2005). The WHO recommended classification of pesticides by hazard and guidelines to classification: 2004. IPCS, WHO, Geneva.

6 Persistent organic pollutants. Available at www.chem.unep.ch/pops/(accessed 28 Feb 2009).

7 Rotterdam Convention. WHO, UNEP, and FAO, Available at www.pic.int.

8 Goldman L, Murray B, Wahlstrom B and Pronczuk J (2004). Childhood pesticide poisoning information for advocacy and action. UNEP, Chatelaine, Switzerland, pp. 26–28.

9 Thundiyil J, Stober J, Besbelli N and Pronczuk J (2008). Acute pesticide poisoning: A proposed classification tool. *Bulletin of the World Health Organization*, 86(3): 161–240.

10 Suk W, Ruchirawat K, Balakrishnan K, Berger M, Carpenter D, Damstra T, Pronczuk J, Koh D, Landrigan P, Makalinao I, Sly P, Xu Y, Zheng B. Environmental threats to children's health in Southeast Asia and the Western Pacific. *Environmental Health Perspectives* **111**(10):1340–1347, 1009.

11 PAHO (2007). Health in the Americas 2007, pp. 236–239, 243. PAHO, WHO, Washington DC,

12 DPR (2009). Summary of results from the California Pesticide Illness Surveillance Program: 2007. DPR, California EPA, Sacramento.

13 Reigart J, Roberts J (1999). *Recognition and Management of Pesticide Poisoning*, 5th ed., pp. 34–47. Washington DC: EPA.

14 ATSDR (2007). *Case Studies in Environmental Medicine: Cholinesterase Inhibitors*. Atlanta: ATSDR, CDC.

15 Jeyaratnam J (1990). Acute pesticide poisoning: A major global health problem. *World Health Statistics Quarterly*, **43**(3):139–144.

16 Eddleston M, Sudarshan K, Senthilkumaran M, Reginald K and Karalliedde L, Senarathna L, de Silva D, Sheriff M, Buckley N, Gunnell D (2006). Patterns of hospital transfer for self-poisoned patients in rural Sri Lanka: Implications for estimating the incidence of self-poisoning in the developing world. *Bulletin of the World Health Organization*, **84**:276–282,.

17 Henao S and Arbelaez M (2002). Epidemiological situation of acute pesticide poisoning in the Central America Isthmus, 1992–2000. *Epidemiology Bulletin*, **23**:5–9.

18 PAHO (2007). Regional Core Health Data Initiative. Washington DC: PAHO, WHO.

19 Kishi M (2002). *Acutely Toxic Pesticides*. Boston, MA: JSI Research and Training Institute

20 McConnell R and Hruska AJ (1993). An epidemic of pesticide poisoning in Nicaragua: Implications for prevention in developing countries. *American Journal of Public Health* **83**:1559–62.

21 Keifer M, McConnell R, Pacheco AF, Daniel W, Rosenstock L (1996). Estimating underreported pesticide poisonings in Nicaragua. *American Journal of Industrial Medicine*, **30**:195–201.

22 Wesseling C, Hogstedt C, Fernandez P and Ahlbom A. (2001). Time trends of occupational pesticide-related injuries in Costa Rica, 1982–1992. *Internationa Journal of Occupational and Environmental Health*, *7*:1–6.

23 Azaroff LS and Neas LM (1999). Acute health effects associated with non-occupational pesticide exposure in rural El Salvador. *Environmental Research* **80**:158–64.

Chapter 9C

Illustrative example C: Lead

David L. Parker and Lisa Ide

Introduction

This section details the extent of hazardous lead exposure and its potential interaction with common nutritional problems. Lead was selected because it has been relatively well studied in the general population. It is meant to serve as a model for the effects of more numerous but less studied substances. These substances include other heavy metals (e.g. mercury) as well as other neurotoxicants (e.g. solvents, pesticides).

Exposure evaluation is complex for children who begin life with an elevated lead body burden reflecting the lead body burden of their mother. The intergenerational effects of child labour may extend to lead exposure if maternal exposure to lead occurs during pregnancy. While not specifically addressed in this review, there is also clear potential for exposure to the developing fetus. This exposure may take place via several routes: mothers working while pregnant, airborne contamination, and contamination of food and water. In almost all circumstances, children are at greater risk than adults [1].

While there are many health effects attributed to lead exposure, this discussion will focus on the neurocognitive changes seen in children primarily because the link with IQ provides a quantitative basis for studies in this field. Lead and other heavy metals are especially toxic to young children and associated with decreased intelligence, impaired neurobehavioural development, growth, and hearing [2]. Nutrition can affect lead levels and so the effects of nutrition are also considered.

The effects of lead on children

The development of the brain and nervous system begins in the early stages of embryonic life and continues through early adulthood. Disruption to this well-organized series of developmental changes will have lasting effects. The developing brain is extremely vulnerable to toxic effects though specific neurodevelopmental data in humans are usually unavailable. However, recent data indicate a negative effect of lead on overall brain growth [3, 4].

Lead exposure in children has been linked to decreased cognitive function and adverse neurobehavioural effects. A meta-analysis of 24 studies of childhood lead exposures related to IQ concludes that lead impairs children's IQ at blood levels under 10 µg/dL [5]. Studies have documented lead exposure and decreased cognitive function from age 24 months through age 10 with decreased scores on the Wechsler Intelligence Scale of 5.8 points for each 10 µg/dL increase in blood lead at age 24 months. This impact persists in early childhood and adolescence [6, 7].

An 11-year follow-up of subjects who had been studied as primary school children showed that those with higher lead levels than their peers had consistently lower IQ scores in fifth grade and subsequently had lower class standing in high school, increased absenteeism, poorer hand–eye coordination and longer reaction times among other neurological findings [8]. Lead exposure in childhood causes decreased intelligence and this effect is present even at low lead levels that are still prevalent in, for example, the United States [9]. A generally agreed upon numerical estimate suggests that for each increase in blood lead of 4 µg/dL, there is a 1 point drop in IQ [10]. Most, if not all data, indicate that lead levels need to be minimized throughout childhood [11].

The effects of lead on delinquent behaviour and antisocial tendencies are equally significant [12, 13]. Even low level lead exposure can have a significant effect on a child's neuropsychological development. As with intelligence, neurobehavioural impact of early childhood lead exposure can persist into high school and beyond. This is confirmed by data from the United States Agency for Toxic Substances and Disease Registries (ATSDR) showing that young adults who had elevated blood lead levels in childhood had poor scores on neurobehavioural tests 15–20 years after their initial exposure [14]. In addition, a health assessment of Idaho residents who lived near a mining and smelting facility demonstrated a dose response relationship with the severity of dysfunction increasing with increasing bone lead concentrations [15].

As more data have become available on the adverse health effects of lead, the acceptable blood lead level has decreased. In 1990, the US Department of Health and Human Services aimed to eliminate blood lead levels greater than 25 µg/dL: the new goal in the United States is to eliminate blood lead levels greater than 10 µg/dL by the year 2010. The threshold level for harmful effects of lead is currently unknown [16].

Occupational exposure of children to lead

Children may be exposed to lead in the production of ceramic pottery, battery recycling, stained glass production, automobile radiator repair, construction, and glassworks. Lead exposure also occurs in the smelting and mining industries and through exposure to fuels [17]. In addition, children's industrial exposures to lead are superimposed on higher environmental exposures seen in developing countries where leaded car fuel is in use [18].

There is, however, almost no information available on toxic occupational exposures in children [17]. Data are lacking on all aspects of this subject: numbers of children exposed, duration of exposure, substances involved, resulting illnesses, and long-term effects. Data are unavailable by country, by region, or globally. There are no accurate data regarding the number of industries around the world that use lead and the total number of people potentially exposed to lead at work. At the time of writing, there are just three reports on lead exposure in children who work. It has been previously noted that 'official data on child labour are generally fragmentary, underestimate informal sector work and family work, and frequently exclude unpaid work' [19].

An observational study of the ceramic tile industry in Victoria, Ecuador describes the local production of roof tiles [20]. Approximately half of the families in this area are involved in producing roof tiles or ceramic objects usually at small work sites situated next to their homes. Clay is extracted from the local mountains and then moulded into tiles or artifacts. The items are glazed with lead salts made from melted batteries. The ceramics are fired in furnaces for 24–48 hours permeating the local air with dust and fumes from both the ceramics and the fuel. No environmental precautions are in place.

Children as young as 6 years were observed working in this trade. Harari and Cullen enrolled 12 children in a cross-sectional evaluation of lead levels [20]. Ten of these children ages 6 to 15 years gave blood samples and lead levels ranged from 23–124 μg/dL with a mean of 70. Three of the children had worked for less than three months; their blood lead levels were < 50 μg/dL. All of the children who had worked longer than three months had blood lead levels greater than 60 μg/dL. Corresponding IQ tests were not done but five of the children had repeated one or more years of school. However, this was a small study and conducted on a convenience sample.

Excessive lead levels have also been observed in child workers in occupations where lead exposure is not traditionally suspected. Children who work as scavengers and street vendors are at risk of hazardous lead exposure. A study of the child scavengers who worked and lived on Smokey Mountain, a garbage dump which received approximately one-third of Manila's garbage before it closed in the 1990s, found that the 20,000 residents were exposed to waste from chemical, hospital, and slaughterhouse sources [21].

Children start scavenging when they are as young as 5 to 7 years old. A 1991 survey of 231 scavengers aged 6 to 15 years found that 68% of boys and 58% of girls had blood lead levels greater than 20 μg/dL. The recorded mean blood lead level was 28.4 μg/dL (standard deviation of 11.5). The authors compared these data to blood samples from 25 school children in metro Manila who had a mean blood lead level of 11 μg/dL [21].

Street vendors are also at risk for lead exposure. A 1993 study of 387 school children and 101 child vendors aged 6 to 14 years in Manila demonstrated that 10% of the school children had blood lead levels in excess of 20 μg/dL as compared to 33% of the street vendors. The mean blood lead level in the street vendors was 17.8 μg/dL [22]. This increased level is most likely secondary to the continued, albeit diminishing use of leaded gasoline in many parts of the world [23].

The effects of nutrition on lead exposure in child labour

Consideration of the effects of toxic exposure in child workers needs to take into account other pertinent public health, economic, and social factors. For example, nutritional status is an important determinant of the impact of lead during early development. Iron-deficiency anaemia is perhaps the most critical micronutrient deficiency related to lead exposure and affects 2 to over 3 billion people worldwide [24, 25].

Epidemiological studies have shown an association between iron deficiency and lead poisoning. Willows and Gray-Donald found evidence of this association among infants with very low blood lead levels (mean = 1.7 μg/dL) [26]. Wright constructed a model predicting that iron-deficient children are more than four times as likely as their iron-replete peers to have blood lead levels >10 μg/dL when tested at a second clinic visit [13].

Of particular concern in considering lead exposure in children is the fact that children are more susceptible to lead toxicity than adults. Children are more vulnerable to absorbed lead than adults because they develop toxicity at lower blood lead levels [27]. Adults absorb 10–15% of lead ingested with meals, however, children and pregnant women can absorb up to 50% [28, 29].

Absorption of lead is even higher in children with low dietary iron, zinc, or calcium intake. Iron deficiency may increase duodenal lead absorption. Low calcium intake activates vitamin D to 1,25 dihydroxyvitamin D causing increased absorption of calcium and lead in intestinal cells [29]. Low zinc intake could be partly responsible for children's increased susceptibility to lead because lead affects zinc-requiring enzymes in the biosynthesis of haem [14].

Iron-deficiency anaemia and other indicators of poor nutrition are associated with poverty [30] as well as race [31]. Child workers in developing countries most often come from poverty-stricken families and would be more likely to suffer from malnutrition and micronutrient deficiencies. The data, however, are limited and conflicting. In the Philippines study of child scavengers, the anaemia rate was 10% compared to the rate of 28% in metro Manila [21]. In a study of male child workers in Jordan, however, 34% of the child workers were found to be anaemic [32]. A study of child workers in Bombay found an anaemia rate of 10% in 73 children in the large slum of Dharavi. The authors speculated that the nutritional status of the Dharavi child workers is better than in 'the great numbers of children elsewhere who do not work but who do not eat' [33].

Determining with any accuracy the extent to which levels of lead in children are related to their occupational exposure is compounded by the lack of separation between the job, home, and the external environment. This lack of distinction is not limited to obvious examples such as child scavengers [34]. Studies unrelated to child labour have documented the risk of toxic exposures to children from contamination in the homes of exposed workers as well as from environmental sources in industrial areas [35].

In the United States, a National Institute of Occupational Safety and Health (NIOSH) case–control study which examined lead exposure in construction workers found significantly higher surface lead concentrations in construction workers' homes than in those of controls [36]. A French study of 125 children with lead-exposed parents found that children's blood levels were significantly higher than the reference group and correlated with their parents' blood lead levels and lead air concentration at their workplace [37]. Environmental contamination affecting children was demonstrated in a study of children from a Chinese village with lead smelters located near the residential area. High concentrations of lead dust were found in the air, soil, on local crops, and on wheat in the farmers' homes. Mean blood lead levels among children were noted to be extremely high [38].

The potential costs of lead exposure to children

A model developed by Landrigan, which relies on the calculations by Salkever, was used to assess the costs of childhood lead poisoning in the United States [39, 40]. The methods used by Landrigan were generalized to form a crude estimate of the magnitude of the problem of lead exposure in child workers. Salkever determined that the loss of 1 IQ point corresponded to an overall reduction in lifetime earnings of 2.4%. Based on the estimate of 4 μg/dL increase in blood lead levels causing a 1 point IQ drop and working on the assumption that there is not a threshold blood lead level for cognitive effects, each 1 μg/dL of blood lead concentration is associated with a decrease in IQ of 0.25.

Table 9C.1 demonstrates the potential IQ decrease in the three cited studies and the subsequent % decrease in lifetime earnings. The potential IQ decrease

Table 9C.1 Estimated earning lost due to lead exposure in child workers

Child workers	Source	Mean blood lead in μg/dL	Potential loss of IQ	Percent decrease in lifetime earnings
Ecuador: ceramic workers	Harari and Cullen, 1995	70.2	17.6	42.1
The Philippines: scavengers	Torres, 1994	28.4	7.1	17.0
The Philippines: street vendors	Martins, 1995	17.8	4.45	10.6

was calculated from the following assumptions: that for each blood lead measurement of 1 μg/dL there is a mean loss of 0.25 IQ points per child and that the loss of 1 IQ point subsequently leads to 2.4% loss of lifetime earnings.

These economic calculations may not accurately estimate the financial costs in developing countries. Moreover, the impact of lead on IQ may vary based on the age of exposure and the acute or chronic nature of the exposure. Another concern is that the lifetime expected earnings calculations from the Philippines and Ecuador come from the average annual income in those counties: salaries the average child worker will not be able to attain for socioeconomic reasons before lead exposure and IQ is taken into account.

Conclusions

The potential magnitude of lead exposure in child workers is considerable. Any definition of hazardous employment needs to include consideration of jobs with potentially toxic occupational exposures. Low levels of many toxicants will effect early brain growth and development and substances such as mercury readily cross the placental barrier or are rapidly absorbed from the intestines of small children [41].

The potential magnitude of the hazard from lead exposure in child workers is, however, unclear, although it is likely that no level of lead exposure can be guaranteed as safe [42]. The remarkable dearth of information dramatically illustrates how toxic occupational exposures in children are overlooked.

In estimating any effect on health from toxins such as lead, the potential for such exposures to interact with pre-existing morbidity such as micronutrient deficiencies should be considered [43, 44]. For example, iron deficiency when combined with elevated levels of lead has been shown to impair neurological development in young children. Because these conditions may be present at the same time, studies focusing on the effect of one should control for the effects of the second. Failure to do so allows for the possibility that, for example, the effect of iron deficiency on cognitive abilities is confounded by unmeasured lead poisoning.

Despite these limitations, several conclusions are quite clear. First, information and research on lead and other toxic occupational exposures in child workers is in its infancy. Second, the magnitude of the problem is potentially immense. Third, additional data will facilitate the capacity of policy makers to determine the types of work that are most detrimental to growth and development. Finally, the potential impact of toxic exposures may manifest in ways that are not traditionally considered by policy makers. This is particularly true if exposure takes place during periods of rapid growth and development or concurrently with other highly prevalent problems such as iron or other micronutrient deficiencies.

Efforts to improve nutritional status and micronutrient replacement are crucial but beyond the scope of this book. Clear policy directives on iron supplementation are necessary because of their importance as a public health problem. Unambiguous distinctions between home and work are recommended to prevent adults from bringing contaminants into the home and to ensure that infants and children are not cared for in locations that are contaminated with toxic materials.

References

1 Firestone MP, Amler RW (2003). Children's environmental health – an international perspective. *International Journal of Hygiene and Environmental Health*, **206**(4–5): 395–400.

2 Koller K, Brown T, Spurgeon A, Levy L (2004). Recent developments in low-level lead exposure and intellectual impairment in children. *Environmental Health Perspectives*, **112**(9):987–94.

3 Cecil KM, Brubaker CJ, Adler CM, Dietrich KN, Altaye M, Egelhoff JC, *et al.* (2008). Decreased brain volume in adults with childhood lead exposure. *PLoS Medicine*, **27**:5(5):e112.

4 Schettler T (2001). Toxic threats to neurologic development of children. *Environmental Health Perspectives*, **109**(Suppl 6):813–6.

5 Needleman HL, Gatsonis CA (1990). Low-level lead exposure and the IQ of children. A meta-analysis of modern studies. *Journal of the American Medical Association*, **2**:263(5)R:673–8.

6 Bellinger DC, Stiles KM, Needleman HL (1992). Low-level lead exposure, intelligence and academic achievement: a long-term follow-up study. *Pediatrics*, **90**(6):855–61.

7 Bellinger D, Sloman J, Leviton A, Rabinowitz M, Needleman HL, Waternaux C (1991). Low-level lead exposure and children's cognitive function in the preschool years. *Pediatrics*, **87**(2):219–27.

8 Needleman HL, Schell A, Bellinger D, Leviton A, Allred EN (1990). The long-term effects of exposure to low doses of lead in childhood. An 11-year follow-up report. *The New England Journal of Medicine*, **322**(2):83–8.

9 Bellinger DC, Needleman HL (2003). Intellectual impairment and blood lead levels. *The New England Journal of Medicine*, **349**(5):500–2

10 Wakefield J (2002). The lead effect? *Environmental Health Perspectives* **110**(10): A574-80.

11 Chen A, Cai B, Dietrich KN, Radcliffe J, Rogan WJ (2007). Lead exposure, IQ, and behavior in urban 5- to 7-year-olds: Does lead affect behavior only by lowering IQ? *Pediatrics*, **119**(3):e650–8.

12 Wigg NR (2001). Low-level lead exposure and children. *Journal of Paediatrics and Child Health*, **37**(5):423–5.

13 Wright RO, Tsaih SW, Schwartz J, Wright RJ, Hu H (2003). Association between iron deficiency and blood lead level in a longitudinal analysis of children followed in an urban primary care clinic. *The Journal of Pediatrics*, **142**(1):9–14.

14 Amler R, Smith L (2001). Achievements in children's environmental health. Atlanta, GA: US Department of Health and Human Services, Agency for Toxic Substances and Disease Registry.

15 Williamson G, Lybarger J, Millete D, Berger-Frank S (2001). Achievements in children's environmental health. In Amler R, Smith L, (eds) *Lasting Neurological Impairment from Lead Exposure in Childhood (A Cohort Study Of Current And Previous Residents of the Silver Valley: Assessment of Lead Exposure and Health Outcomes)*, pp. 54–5. Atlanta: ATSDR.

16 Meyer PA, Pivetz T, Dignam TA, Homa DM, Schoonover J, Brody D (2003). Surveillance for elevated blood lead levels among children – United States, 1997–2001. *MMWR Surveillence Summary* **52**(10):1–21.

17 Woolf AD (2002). Health hazards for children at work. *Journal of Toxicology*, **40**(4):477–82.

18 Donohoe M (2003). Correspondence. *New Engl and Journal of Medicine*, **349**:501.

19 Heynman JE (2003). *Global Inequalities at Work: Work's impact on the Health of Individuals, Families, and Societies.* New York: Oxford University Press.

20 Harari R, Cullen MR (1995). Childhood lead intoxication associated with manufacture of roof tiles and ceramics in the Ecuadorian Andes. *Archives of Environmental Health*, **50**(5):393.

21 Torres E, Subida R, Rabuco L (1994). Health profile of child scavengers in Smokey Mountain, Balut, Tondo, Manila: German Agency for Technical Cooperation/ International Labor Organization/College of Public Health, University of the Philippines Manila.

22 Martins J (1995). Philippines environmental health assessment: an agenda for action. Unpublished manuscript.

23 Meyer PA, Brown MJ, Falk H (2008). Global approach to reducing lead exposure and poisoning. *Mutation Research*. **659**(1–2):166–75.

24 Zimmermann MB, Hurrell RF (2007). Nutritional Iron Deficiency. *Lancet*, **370**(9586):511–20.

25 Lynch S, Stoltzfus R, Rawat R (2007). Critical review of strategies to prevent and control iron deficiency in children. Food and nutrition bulletin, **28**(Suppl 4):S610–20.

26 Willows ND, Gray-Donald K (2002). Blood lead concentrations and iron deficiency in Canadian aboriginal infants. *Science of the Total Environment*, **289**(1–3):255–60.

27 Agency for Toxic Substances and Disease Registry A (1999). Toxicological profile for lead. Atlanta, GA. US: Department of Health and Human Services. Public Health Service.

28 Timbrell J (2002). *Introduction to Toxicology*. New York and London: Taylor & Francis.

29 Wigle D (2003). *Child Health and the Environment*. New York: Oxford University Press.

30 Wadsworth M (2000). Early Life. In Marmot M, Wilkinson RG (eds), *Social Determinants of Health*. Oxford: Oxford University Press.

31 Brotanek JM, Gosz J, Weitzman M, Flores G (2007). Iron deficiency in early childhood in the United States: risk factors and racial/ethnic disparities. *Pediatrics*, **120**(3): 568–75.

32 Hawamdeh H, Spencer N (2001). Work, family socioeconomic status, and growth among working boys in Jordan. *Archives of Disease in Childhood*, **84**(4):311-4.

33 Mehta MN, Prabhu SV, Mistry HN (1985). Child labor in Bombay. *Child Abuse and Neglect*, **9**(1):107–11.

34 Landrigan PJ (2002). The worldwide problem of lead in petrol. *Bulletin of the World Health Organization*, **80**(10):768.

35 Knishkowy B, Baker EL (1986). Transmission of occupational disease to family contacts. *American Journal of Industrial Medicine*, **9**(6):543–50.

36 Piacitelli GM, Whelan EA, Sieber WK, Gerwel B (1997). Elevated lead contamination in homes of construction workers. *American Industrial Hygiene Association Journal*, **58**(6):447–54.

37 Laforest L, Annino MC, Alluard A, Precausta D, van den Wiele F, Albouy J, *et al.* (1999). [Epidemiologic study of lead contamination of children of occupationally exposed parents]. *Revue d'epidemiologie et de sante publique*, **47**(5): 433–41.

38 Wu Y, Huang Q, Zhou X, Hu G, Wang Z, Li H, *et al.* (2002) Study on the effects of lead from small industry of battery recycling on environment and children's health. *Zhonghua liu xing bing xue za zhi = Zhonghua liuxingbingxue zazhi*, **23**(3): 167–71.

39 Landrigan PJ, Schechter CB, Lipton JM, Fahs MC, Schwartz J (2002). Environmental pollutants and disease in American children: estimates of morbidity, mortality, and costs for lead poisoning, asthma, cancer, and developmental disabilities. *Environmental Health Perspectives*, **110**(7):721–8.

40 Salkever DS (1995). Updated estimates of earnings benefits from reduced exposure of children to environmental lead. *Environmental Research*, **70**(1):1–6.

41 Wallinga D (2004). Preventing pollution protects children. *Healthy Generations*, **4**:8–9.

42 Bellinger DC (2008). Very low lead exposures and children's neurodevelopment. *Current Opinion in Pediatrics*, **20**(2):172–7.

43 Clark M, Royal J, Seeler R (1988). Interaction of iron deficiency and lead and the hematologic findings in children with severe lead poisoning. *Pediatrics*, **81**(2):247–54.

44 Mahaffey KR, Annest JL (1986). Association of erythrocyte protoporphyrin with blood lead level and iron status in the second National Health and Nutrition Examination Survey, 1976–1980. *Environmental Research*, **41**(1):327–38.

Chapter 9D

Illustrative example D: Silicosis and silicotuberculosis

Raheela Ayub and David L. Parker

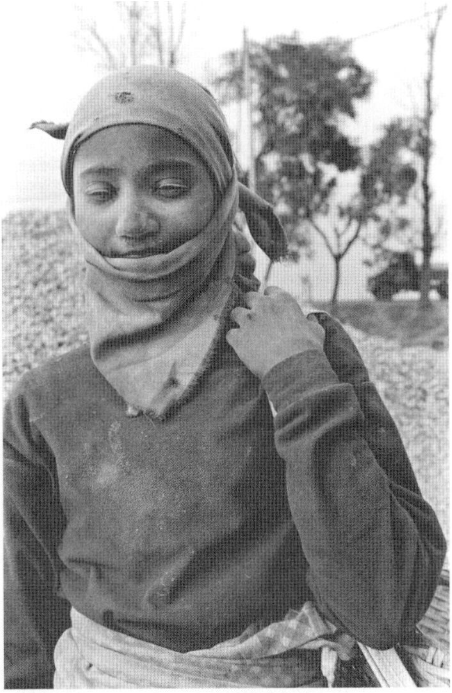

Stone quarry worker, Nepal

Introduction

Silica exposure occurs during activities that involve crushing stone; repairing or constructing roads; making pottery, glass, and bricks; mining, blacksmithing, and carving stone. The inhalation and deposition of respirable crystalline silica is a common occupational exposure resulting in silicosis, a fibrotic disease (scarring) of the upper regions of the lungs [1]. In general, silicosis arises at least a decade or more following the onset of exposure.

Tuberculosis (TB) is caused by the bacteria *Mycobacterium tuberculosis*. TB is spread when infected individuals are in close contact with others. Although the organism can cause disease throughout the body, it is associated most frequently with lung infections. [1]. TB remains one of the leading causes of mortality around the world.

Among adults, a well-established link exists between silicosis and TB (i.e., silicotuberculosis) as well as other mycobacterial diseases [2]. Silicotuberculosis provides an example of why the evaluation of exposure and subsequent illness is critical to understanding the potential long-term effect of work on children and communities.

Compelling evidence demonstrates that silicotuberculosis: (1) is likely to be a highly prevalent problem because of how commonly children work in the dusty trades listed above, (2) affects young workers as they enter the third decade of life, and (3) impacts large segments of the community if they are not adequately treated.

Silicosis

Silicosis is caused by exposure to crystalline silica (quartz). Crystalline silica is found in nearly every mineral deposit. Exposure to silica is associated with the development of silicosis and other diseases. This chapter does not discuss other silica-associated illnesses such as lung cancer, chronic obstructive pulmonary disease, and autoimmune illnesses.

Three types of silicosis may develop: (1) chronic silicosis, which usually occurs after 10 or more years of exposure at relatively low levels of dust (this represents the vast majority of silicosis cases), (2) accelerated silicosis, which develops 5 to 10 years after the first exposure, or (3) acute silicosis, which develops after exposure to high concentrations of respirable crystalline silica and results in symptoms from a few weeks to 5 years after the first exposure [2]. In the remainder of this essay, silicosis refers to chronic silicosis.

Silicosis is characterized by the formation of nodules in the upper part of the lungs and surrounding lymph nodes. Initially, shortness of breath is present only with exertion. As the disease progresses, individuals develop cough, sputum production, and shortness of breathe at rest [3].

The risk of silicosis increases with increased intensity of exposure, with duration of exposure, or both [4]. Studies of gold miners in South Africa, granite quarry workers in Hong Kong, metal ore miners in the United States, and coal miners in Scotland, have shown that chronic silicosis may develop or progress even after exposure to silica has ended [2]. Hence, there is no guarantee that removing a worker from exposure will stop silicosis from developing or progressing [2]. This is particularly relevant for young workers, who have many more years to develop illness than adult workers.

Globally, there are no good estimates on the prevalence or incidence of silicosis. Reports of silicosis from the World Health Organization stem from different time periods. Although the authors solicited input from experts around the world, we were not able to find up-to-date statistics on the global prevalence and incidence of silicosis in adults, let alone children [5]. The magnitude of the problem among adult workers in China, Vietnam, Brazil, Canada, Columbia, and the United States, among others, indicates a serious and persistent problem among both old and young workers.

No studies have been located regarding the extent of silica exposure among working children. However, an examination of available data on dusty occupations common to children such as mining, brick making, and foundry work showed a high risk of silicosis within each category [6–8] These studies are reviewed below under the discussion of silicotuberculosis.

Tuberculosis

M. tuberculosis may cause either latent or active illness. Active disease is present when a person has clinical symptoms (e.g. cough, shortness of breath) and signs of TB (e.g. X-ray findings). With latent disease, there are no signs or symptoms of the illness; rather, the body harbours the bacteria that could become active if immunity were to weaken. The diagnosis of latent TB can be made with purified protein derivative (PPD) skin test [1].

In 2007, the global incidence of TB was estimated at 9.3 million cases. The disease was responsible for 1.3 million deaths in people without HIV and 456,000 deaths among people with HIV [9]. In the same year, there were an estimated 511,000 cases of multi-drug resistant TB, or about 4.9% of new and previously treated cases [9]. Globally, TB was the 7th leading cause of death and is projected to remain at this level into the foreseeable future [10]. In countries with a high incidence of TB, children have up to a 50% risk of infection when exposed to adults with active disease [11].

Risk factors for tuberculosis among working children

It can be reasonably surmised that young workers are at increased risk of both latent and active TB for several reasons:

(1) A high prevalence of TB is found in many countries that have the highest numbers of young workers.

(2) Young workers frequently live in poor and often crowded communities.

(3) Nutritional deficiencies are associated with opportunistic infections such as TB [12]. These risk factors are correlated (i.e. poverty leads to poor nutrition and crowding). A complete discussion of this topic is beyond the scope of this book.

The relationship between poverty and TB has repeatedly been demonstrated in studies around the world. When compared with wealthier individuals, poverty imparts an increased risk of TB that ranges from approximately 50% to just under six-fold. Crowding appears to impart a three- to five-fold increased risk of disease [13–18]. TB is also correlated with poor nutrition. However, it is difficult to ascertain if poor nutrition is a risk factor for disease, an outcome of active illness, or both [1, 19–22]. In addition, young workers in some regions of the world are at increased risk of HIV/AIDS, another risk factor for TB [23].

Silicosis and tuberculosis

Silicotuberculosis occurs when the lungs' defense mechanisms are overwhelmed by silica dust and are unable to kill *M. tuberculosis* [2]. According to the United States National Institute for Occupational Safety and Health (NIOSH), 'the association between TB and silicosis has been firmly established'.[2] Increased risk of TB has been repeatedly demonstrated in surveillance, case–control, and cohort studies from around the world. This increased risk ranges from approximately two- to ten-fold when compared with the general population [24–28].

Saiyed *et al.* [29] studied workers in small-scale potteries in India. Many had started working in their late teens. Within this industry, the grinding and mixing of raw materials generates large amounts of dust. The highest levels of respirable dust were up to nine times the permissible exposure levels in the United States. Overall, 15% (n=44) of workers showed evidence of silicosis on X-ray. A similar number had radiographic findings of TB. However, workers in the dustiest areas had a prevalence of silicosis of 31% and a prevalence of TB of 27%.

Chien *et al.* evaluated silicosis among Vietnamese brick workers. Disease prevalence was as high as 18% for long-term workers. Exposure was up to five times the permissible exposure level in the United States. While brickwork is a common occupation for children, children were not present in this study. A study of 195 foundry workers in India found a prevalence of silicosis of 27% and a prevalence of TB of 10%. Of those with silicosis, 15% had silicotuberculosis. Among the workers, 35 were 15 to 24 years old, with one worker in this age group having TB [31].

Conclusions

Despite the well-documented risk of TB among those with silicosis, diagnosis and treatment is problematic. First, recovery of the TB organism is difficult because of the presence of scarring in the lungs [29]. Second, as rates of HIV increase in developing nations, testing for TB may give false negative results [32]. Third, for those in poverty, the ability to get and afford treatment is, at best, difficult and, at times, entirely absent [33–35]. Treatment should be vigorous, carefully monitored, and longer than for uncomplicated TB [3].

The authors were unable to locate studies that correlated the prevalence of silicosis with either the prevalence or incidence of TB on a global basis. The absence of data is an important problem that has not been well addressed. Conservatively, if exposed workers with silicosis experience a five-fold (mid-range estimate) increase in risk when compared with the general population, the risk of silicotuberculosis in some regions of the world is likely to be extremely high. For example, in some regions of the India, the TB notification rate for new illness and relapse is 120 to 245 cases per 100,000 per year [36].

Because there is no treatment for silicosis, prevention is key [1]. Epidemiological studies suggest that the estimated risk of silicosis for a 45-year working lifetime is 47 to 90% for concentrations equal to the current United States Occupational Safety and Health (OSHA) Permissible Exposure Level (PEL) [2].

Control measures include dust control, process enclosure and isolation of dusty-producing activities, and good ventilation. While personal protective equipment may offer some level of protection, this is expensive, rarely available, and never suited to the needs of children.

Work in many common occupations places children at risk of exposure to silica and the development of silicosis. However, the discussion of hazardous work often takes place without serious consideration of risks that work imparts on the community and vice versa. The problem of silicotuberculosis is a serious public health hazard. The risk of TB rises substantially among workers who develop silicosis. This increased risk occurs in communities that are already likely to be at high risk and where resources may not be adequate to assure diagnosis and treatment.

While not the subject of this chapter, the absence of data on the incidence and prevalence of silicosis and silicotuberculosis among children and adults points to the need for a global surveillance programme. It is likely that this would provide important data on a preventable cause of morbidity and mortality.

References

1 Balmes J (2007). Occupational Lung Diseases. In *Current Occupational & Environmental Medicine*, Ladou J, 4th Edition. McGraw-Hill: San Francisco, California, USA.

2 NIOSH (2002). Review of health effects of occupational exposure to respirable crystalline silica. Cincinnati, OH: U.S. Department of Health and Human Services, Public Health Service, Centers for Disease Control, National Institute for Occupational Safety and Disease, Publications no 2002-129.

3 Levin S, Lilis R (1998). Silicosis. In: *Maxcy-Rosenau-Last Public Health & Preventive Medicine*, Wallace R, Doebbeling B, Last J, 14th Edition. McGraw-Hill: Stamford, Connecticut, USA.

4 teWaterNaude JM, Ehrlich RI, Churchyard *et al.* (2006). Tuberculosis and silica exposure in South African gold miners, *Occupational and Environmental Medicine*, **63**:187–92.

5 World Health Organization. *Silicosis*. Available at http://www.who.int/mediacentre/factsheets/fs238/en/ (accessed 17 July 2009).

6 Saiyed, HN, Parikh DJ, Ghodasara NB *et al.* (1985). Silicosis in slate pencil workers: I. An environmental and medical study. *American Journal of Industrial Medicine*, **8**: 127–33.

7 Samal RK, Reddaiah VP, Mukhopadhyay S, Nath LM (1986). Prevalence of pulmonary tuberculosis among iron foundry workers. *Indian Journal of Industrial Medicine*, **32**: 116–20.

8 Chien VC, Chai SK, Hai DN *et al.* (2002). Pneumoconiosis among workers in a Vietnamese refractory brick facility. *American Journal of Industrial Medicine*, **42**(5):397–402.

9 World Health Organization. *Global Tuberculosis Control*. Available at http://www.who.int/tb/publications/global_report/2009/pdf/full_report.pdf

10 Lopez AD, Murray CC (1998). The global burden of disease, 1990–2020. *Nature Medicine*, **4**:1241–3;

11 Michaud CM, Murray CJ, Bllom BR (2001). Burden of disease – implications for future research. *Journal of the American Medical Association*, **285**:535–9.

12 Nakoaka H, Lawson L, Bertel Squire S, *et al.* (2006). Risk for tuberculosis among children. *Emerging Infectious Diseases*, **12**:1383–8.

13 Oguntibeju OO, Van den Heever WM, Van Schalkwyk FE (2007). The interrelationship between nutrition and the immune system in HIV infection: A review. *Pakistan Journal of Biological Sciences*, **10**(24):4327–38

14 Muniyandi M, Ramachandran R (2008). Socioeconomic inequalities of tuberculosis in India, *Expert Opinion on Pharmacotherapy*, **9**(10):1623–8.

15 Geraldes Santos Mde L, Figueiredo Vendramini SH, Gazetta CE, Cruz Oliveira SA, Scatena Villa TC (2007). Poverty: socioeconomic characterization at tuberculosis, *Revista Latino-Americana de Enfermagem*, **15** Spec. No: 762-7.

16 Vendramini SH, Santos ML, Gazetta CE, Chiaravalloti-Neto F, Ruffino-Netto A, Villa TC (2006). Tuberculosis risks and socio-economic level: A case study of a city in the Brazilian south-east, 1998–2004. *International Journal of Tuberculosis and Lung Disease*, **10**(11):1231–5.

17 Coker R, McKee M, Atun R, Dimitrova B *et al.* (2006) Risk factors for pulmonary tuberculosis in Russia: Case–control study. *British Medical Journal*, **332**(7533):85–7.

18 Hill PC, Jackson-Sillah D, donkor SA, Out J, Adegbola RA, Lienhardt C (2006). Risk factors for pulmonary tuberculosis: A clinic-based case control study in The Gambia. *BMC Public Health*, **19**(6):156.

19 Tomee S, Kaewkungwal J, Fungladda W, Silachamroon W, Akarasewi P, Sunakorn P (2005). The association between environmental factors and tuberculosis infection among household contacts. *Southeast Asian Journal of Tropical Medicine and Public Health*, **36**(Suppl 4):222–4.

20 Pakasi TA, Karyadi E, Domans WM, van der Meer JW, van der Valden K (2009). Malnutrition and socio-demographic factors associated with pulmonary tuberculosis in Timor and Rote Islands, Indonesia. *International Journal of Tuberculosis and Lung Disease*, **13**(6):755–9.

21 Karyadi E, Schultink W, Nelwan RH *et al.* (2000). Poor micronutrient status of active pulmonary tuberculosis patients in Indonesia. *Journal of Nutrition*, **130**(12):2953–8.

22 Sasidharan PK, Rajeev E, Vijayakumari V (2002). Tuberculosis and vitamin D deficiency. *Journal of Association of Physicians of India*, **50**:554–8.

23 Metcalfe N (2005). A study of tuberculosis, malnutrition and gender in Sri Lanka. *Transactions of Royal Society of Tropical Medicine and Hygiene*, **99**(2):115–9.

24 Mulenga EM, Miller HB, Sinkala T, Hysong TA, Burgess JL (2005). Silicosis and tuberculosis in Zambian miners. *International Journal of Occupational and Environmental Health*, **11**(3):259–62.

25 Althouse RB, Bang KM, Castellan RM (1995). Tuberculosis comortality with silicosis – United States, 1979–1991. *Applied Occupational and Environmental Hygiene*, **10**(12):1037–41.

26 Corbett EL, Churchyard GJ, Clayton T, Herselman P, Williams B, Hayes R, Mulder D, De Cock KM (1999). Risk factors for pulmonary mycobacterial disease in South African gold miners. *American Journal of Respiratory and Critical Care Medicine*, **159**:94–9.

27 Sherson D, Lander F (1990). Morbidity of pulmonary tuberculosis among silicotic and nonsilicotic foundry workers in Denmark. *Journal of Occupational Medicine*, **32**(2):110–13.

28 Cowie RL (1994). The epidemiology of tuberculosis in gold miners with silicosis. *American Journal of Respiratory and Critical Care Medicine*, **150**:1460–2.

29 Davies JCA (2001). Silicosis and tuberculosis among South African gold miners – An overview of recent studies and current issues. *South African Medical Journal*, **91**: 562–6.

30 Saiyed HN, Ghodasara NB, Sathwara NG, Patel GC, Parikh DJ, Kashyap SK (1995). Dustiness, silicosis and tuberculosis in small scale pottery workers, *Indian Journal of Medical Research*, **102**:138–42.

31 Chien VC, Chai SK, Hai DN *et al.* (2002). Pneumoconiosis among workers in a Vietnamese refractory brick facility. *American Journal of Industrial Medicine*, **42**(5):397–402.

32 Samal RK. Reddaiah VP, Mukhopadhyay S, Nath LM (1986). Prevalence of pulmonary tuberculosis among iron foundry workers. *Indian Journal of Industrial Medicine*, **32**: 116–20.

33 ATS (American Thoracic Society) (1997). Adverse effects of crystalline silica exposure. *American Journal of Respiratory and Critical Care Medicine*, **155**:761–768.

34 Mahmoudi A, Iseman M (1993). Pitfalls in the care of patients with tuberculosis. *Journal of the American Medical Association*, **270**:265–8.

35 Brudney K, Dobkin J (1991). Resurgent tuberculosis in New York City. *American Review of Respiratory Diseases*, **144**:745–9.

36 Combs DL, O'Brien RJ, Ctiter LJ (1990). USPHS TB short-course chemotherapy trial 21: Effectiveness, toxicity, and acceptability. The report of final results. *Annals of Internal Medicine*, **112**:397–406.

37 World Health Organization. Country Profile: India Available at http://apps.who.int/globalatlas/predefinedReports/TB/PDF_Files/ind.pdf (accessed 21 October 2009).

Chapter 9E

Illustrative example E: HIV and AIDS

Anita Amorim and Nadine Osseiran

Introduction

In their 2008 Annual Report 'Towards Universal Access', UNAIDS estimated that as of mid-2008 an estimated global total of 33 million (30.6–36.1 million) people were living with HIV. In 2007, an estimated 2.7 million (2.2–3.2 million) individuals were newly infected and 2.0 million (1.8–2.3 million) died of AIDS-related illnesses. Sub-Saharan Africa has been the region most severely affected: an estimated 22.0 million (20.5–23.6 million) people living with HIV, or 67% of the global total live in sub-Saharan Africa. Almost one-third of all new HIV infections and AIDS-related deaths worldwide occur in this region. Patterns of infection in Africa differ from those around the world. Women account for 60% or more of new HIV infections in sub-Saharan Africa; in other regions men represent the majority of new infections and of people living with HIV. Globally, across all populations, adolescents and young adults are most likely to be exposed to HIV [1].

The HIV epidemic has had significant economic and social repercussions, including in the labour market. It has forced many young people and children who are HIV-positive, orphaned or having sick relatives, to enter the labour market prematurely. In Uganda for example, where HIV prevalence reached 5.4% in 2007 (UNAIDS, 2008), there are an estimated 2.5 million children between 7 and 14 years engaged in economic activities; among them 1.4 million children who are aged less than 12 years [2].

This chapter explores the impact of HIV on education and child labour with particular focus on some special groups and considers the impact of initiatives to tackle HIV in the particular context of its effect on child labour.

Impact of HIV on Child Labour

Although it cuts across socioeconomic groups, the transmission of HIV follows long established inequality pathways that intensified in late 20th century [3]. The relationship between poverty and HIV is bi-directional.

Poverty places people in situations where they face higher risks of HIV infection, such as the migration to find employment or income. In turn, HIV infection itself becomes a major financial drain on households, communities, businesses, and countries, which in turn leads to greater poverty.

Across sub-Saharan Africa, in response to socio-economic development patterns, millions of people have migrated to secure employment. Plantations, mines, and industries have secured massive quantities of labour, largely drawn from the countryside. The increasing concentration of both formal and informal sector employment in urban centres has also drawn millions of young people into the cities [4]. The combination of being far away from regular sexual partners, living in the context of different social norms, lacking adequate recreational facilities, and the use of alcohol and drugs contribute to a higher risk of HIV infection in migrant workers.

Households that are affected by HIV experience dramatic cuts in income. The household impact begins as soon as a member of the household starts to suffer from HIV-related illnesses. To supplement this economic loss, children may drop out of school and work. Girls and boys who work commonly contribute about 20–25% towards family income (there is little systematic evidence on this, but for research and study, this is a general assumption that is made and adopted in the ILO/IPEC study 'Investing in every child: An economic study of the costs and benefits of eliminating child labour', International Labour Office, International Programme on the Elimination of Child Labour (IPEC), Geneva, 2003; other references are: Rau, Bill, 'Globalization, HIV/AIDS and child labour' (draft), 26 May 2001, and UNICEF, 'Armed conflict, HIV/AIDS and child labour in Uganda', (Government of Uganda – UNICEF Country Programme 2001–2005, p. 4).

Initially, most children seek work based upon their parents' experiences. So for example, children whose parents worked on a commercial agricultural estate are likely to find employment on the same estate. A growing number of children affected by HIV, however, find work in the informal sector in urban areas [6, 7].

The effect of HIV on education and schooling

HIV infection affects both the uptake and availability of schooling. It reduces the number of children in school, especially girls. The increased costs of care for HIV-affected family members also reduce any household capacity to meet even the most modest of educational expenses.

In countries with a high prevalence of HIV, there are severe constraints on the capacity and capability to provide educational services. In some cases there are high levels of morbidity and mortality among teachers. UNICEF has estimated that in 1999, 860,000 children in sub-Saharan Africa lost their teachers to AIDS [8]. In Zambia, teacher deaths doubled from 680 in 1996, to 1300 in the first 10 months of 1998. Whilst not all of these deaths can be attributed to AIDS, the number of teacher deaths in 1998 represented a mortality rate about 70% higher than the mortality rate in the general population. For the education system, the 1998 deaths were equivalent to the loss of about two-thirds of the annual output of newly trained teachers from all training institutions combined [9].

Many teachers also find that they are now called upon to provide psychosocial support to pupils to help them deal with the stresses arising from HIV at home. These HIV-related stresses which teachers experience, in the classroom and at home, need to be acknowledged in teacher training. It has also been suggested that some male teachers have used their status and income to obtain sex with school children and women of less secure means in surrounding communities and teachers [9].

In the face of these pressures, education itself remains an important tool for preventing the spread of HIV infection. People who have had the benefit of education are less likely to expose themselves to the risk of infection. The education sector has an existing infrastructure which can be used for HIV education. Teachers, however, need to be appropriately trained to deal with the consequences of HIV infection in their pupils and their families. In response to this problem, the Zambian Ministry of Education has proposed the introduction of HIV/AIDS counselling for teachers and other education personnel and the integration of HIV/AIDS awareness into its in-service training programmes [9].

Special groups

Some groups of children merit special consideration in the context of the HIV and child labour. These include: (a) orphans due to AIDS; (b) children living with HIV or at risk of HIV due to the nature of their work, and (c) girls, who are at increased risk due to gender inequalities.

Orphans due to AIDS

Children under the age of 15 years who have lost one or both their parents due to AIDS are termed orphans due to AIDS. The gender of the parent who has died from AIDS plays an important role in determining which children in the family work and the type of work they undertake [10]. When an adult falls ill or dies, one or more children may be sent away to be cared for by extended-family members. As the number of orphans has grown and the number of care-givers has reduced, traditional community coping mechanisms have been stretched to breaking point. While grandmothers are most likely to take in orphans, they are also likely to be poor and unable to offer substantive material support for children, especially as they themselves reach the age of retirement. In some cases relatives may refuse to take on responsibility for additional child care, or many of those who take responsibility may be unable to look after the children properly [11, 12].

A child remaining at home may therefore take on a parental role or even become the head of the household. These children and their siblings may then drop out of school and enter the labour market. In patrilineal societies, widows and their children risk losing household assets and any claims to land or livestock [13]. Even where legislation provides for the inheritance of assets, cultural practices may take precedent. Children orphaned by HIV may therefore have no assets to bring to caretakers, for example to pay for their education. Many orphaned children are stigmatized and suffer both direct and indirect discrimination. Stigma and discrimination reduce the opportunities for education, job training, and decent work for youth. These children may then take on the worst forms of child labour.

Studies suggest that on becoming an AIDS orphan, the likelihood of a child attending school is reduced by 50% [14]. Orphans also face an increased longer-term risk of stunting and malnourishment [15]. Orphans who do continue to attend school spend less time in school than they did prior to losing a parent. Many orphans are unable to pay school fees and never complete basic schooling. Even when basic education is free, children may not go to school if they cannot afford to buy uniforms and other scholastic materials.

Children living with HIV or at risk of HIV due to the nature of their work

Children may contract HIV from their mother, or through exposure to HIV infection through child labour. Child labour activities that expose children to sexual abuse or the use of drugs and alcohol place children at a particularly high risk of HIV infection. These include, for example, children in commercial sex exploitation, children affected by war, child domestic labourers, and street children [16].

Many adults seek out children for commercial sex because of a perception that there is less danger of HIV infection. There is also a common myth that younger girls can 'disinfect' a person who is HIV-positive. Children subjected to commercial sexual exploitation are at risk of early pregnancy and maternal mortality, sexually transmitted diseases including HIV, and physical, psychological, and emotional abuse [17].

Trafficking of children for sexual exploitation is on the increase due to increased demand, including from tourists. However, there is less available evidence of sexual exploitation in African countries when compared with Asia.

Although commercial and survival sex are extensive in sub-Saharan Africa, sexual exchanges occur more frequently in less formalized settings when compared to Asia, making data collection more difficult [18].

The International Labour Organization International Programme on the Elimination of Child Labour (ILO/IPEC) has undertaken a series of rapid assessments that have shown the links between HIV and child labour. An ILO/IPEC Rapid Assessment of 250 children in prostitution found that poverty, a lack of education, and poor employment opportunities for youth, especially in girls, were associated with child prostitution [19]. Being orphaned was associated with children getting involved in commercial sexual exploitation. The children in the study were often illiterate or semi-literate and 20% of the respondents indicated that they could not find any other job as a result of their poor literacy. There was little use of condoms: 54% of girls said that they did not use condoms regularly and 68% reported that clients refused to use condoms. The majority of the children started prostitution between the ages of 10 and 13 years. Health care was a problem and 95% of the girls stated that clients and the police repressed, beat, and raped them. About 10% of all those interviewed showed signs of HIV-related illness and all had children.

Girls at increased risk due to gender inequalities

Gender inequalities are a major driving force behind the HIV epidemic. In the worst-affected African countries, the highest levels of new infections are found among women and girls. Women in the age group of 15–49 years represent 43% of all new HIV infections [1]. Girls are most vulnerable to HIV due to their ascribed role in the family and society.

Low social and economic status, a relative lack of education amongst girls and certain exploitative working sectors increase the vulnerability of women and girls to HIV. Girls are more likely to be victims of commercial sexual exploitation, which poses great risks. Social norms and the attributes and roles that some societies ascribe to women may deny them knowledge of sexual health practices and prevent them from controlling their own sexual health. Financial pressures stemming from HIV may result in poor families taking their daughters rather than their sons out of school. The financial returns from labour in girls are perceived to exceed the anticipated return from education. Girls are also often considered to have more capability than boys in providing care to HIV-positive relatives at home [20].

Reversing the spread of HIV and its effects on child labour therefore requires that women's rights are realized. The gender dimension of HIV has been recognized in the ILO Code of Practice on HIV/AIDS and the World of Work [21] and in the Resolution on Women, the Girl Child and HIV/AIDS adopted by the UN Commission on the Status of Women [22].

Initiatives to address HIV-induced child labour

Numerous programmes and initiatives have been developed to support children affected by HIV, but few have sought to address the socioeconomic factors driving the pandemic. Little has been done to develop and implement policies or legislation aimed at reducing the likelihood of children affected by HIV from being drawn into child labour.

In 2001 therefore the ILO, through its International Programme on the Elimination of Child Labour (IPEC) sought to develop a programme to address the issues of child labour and HIV. A number of ILO supported studies and workshops on the prevention of HIV-induced child labour were followed by the elaboration of a plan of action to combat HIV-induced child labour at a workshop in Lusaka in 2003 [23].

An ILO/IPEC pilot project (2004–2008) was put in place to prevent and combat HIV-induced child labour in sub-Saharan Africa with funding from the United States Department of Labour (USDOL) [24]. Building on the capacity of national partner organizations in Uganda and Zambia, the project developed community-based models for the prevention of HIV affected boys and girls dropping out of school and entering child labour, and for the withdrawal of those already engaged in the worst forms of child labour. This project put in place specific strategies to address HIV-induced child labour at national and local levels. It developed models of intervention that put in place referrals to education and training, and offered scholastic materials, vocational training, health and psychosocial counseling, and support for reintegration of working children into communities. In an effort to ensure sustainability, the project set up community structures and social protection schemes for HIV-affected families. These included income-generating activities and savings schemes. These pilot models are available for replication in other countries.

The project also supported the Governments of Uganda and Zambia to develop and implement policies and programmes to address HIV and child labour. IPEC worked with employers' and workers' organizations in both countries to raise awareness on HIV and child labour. IPEC also developed tools for policy makers and programme planners to facilitate the spread of good practices, which were shared with several other countries in the continent.

Over 5000 HIV affected boys and girls in Uganda and Zambia have been recipients of the project and over 500 HIV affected families have benefited from income-generating activity schemes and/or savings schemes. The project has also supported the Governments in Uganda and Zambia in mainstreaming HIV into National Child Labour Policies. In November 2006 in Uganda a National Child Labour Policy was adopted with a targeted impact on implementation on over 1.5 million boys and girls affected by HIV/AIDS [25].

The project has also sought to increase the awareness of HIV-induced child labour issues through a media campaign. Several tools, such as manuals and initiatives for teachers, organizations working on child labour, policy makers and planners have been developed and tested and subsequently disseminated to and used in other countries, such as in Kenya, Ghana, Senegal, Cameroon, Tanzania, Malawi, Madagascar, South Africa, and Botswana. Some of these child labour tools have also been translated and disseminated in Asia.

Government, employers' and workers' organizations and civil society organizations in Uganda and Zambia continue in their struggle against child labour and HIV-induced child labour. The capacities of these groups and organizations to fight HIV-induced child labour have been increased as a result of this work. New models of practice and interventions are now used in an effort to sustain these efforts and to ensure that child labour is included in new policies and plans to address the HIV pandemic.

Conclusions

The millions of adults of working age who have and continue to lose their lives as a result of HIV and AIDS have left a major gap in national workforces. If unchecked this gap will continue to call on children to fill roles previously held by adults. HIV has placed millions of children in situations where they are likely to have to work more and at an earlier age, often without the benefits of adequate education or training. There has also been increased demand for younger children within the sex industry.

An estimated 15 million AIDS orphans (in 2007) will enter the workforce with many disadvantages: gaps in education, limited technical skills, psychological problems associated with the loss of a parent and the stigma and discrimination that come with that [16]. In addition there is a severe lack of social support structures and pressures on traditional extended family and community support. These children are not the first choice for the formal and more regulated sector such as some manufacturing, finance/insurance, or public service but are more likely to end up working in informal and unregulated agriculture, manufacturing, sales, and services.

The implications for all forms of child labour are, however, likely to be mixed. With most children affected by HIV unable to gain quality education or training, there is limited scope for moving into existing positions. Also, as business productivity, competitiveness, and profitability are compromised by HIV in the workforce, many businesses will be unable to hire new employees and will therefore offer reduced tax returns to governments, which might have been used for training and employment creation. Poor economic performance decreases public spending on the social sector, just at the time when social support services are most needed [26]. For children affected by HIV or at risk of infection, the labour market does not offer short-term hope for achieving economic security.

The HIV pandemic in sub-Saharan Africa is the crisis of a generation. The response from government, non-governmental organizations, the private and the informal sector needs to expand on all fronts; health, social, and economic. Whilst in prevention lies the hope of stopping AIDS, the lives of the current generation of children and the next depend upon the support and protection that society can offer them [27]. The solution to the current situation of HIV-induced child labour depends upon the effective management of the poverty induced by the epidemic with mitigation strategies to address the already affected girls and boys and their households. International organizations, governments, employers' and workers' organizations, non-governmental organizations, the private and the informal sector, and households and individuals all have a role to play; but there is a need for much greater coordination in working towards a common objective.

Acknowledgements

The authors wish to thank the following people who supported this contribution: Akky de Kort, Chief Technical Advisor, ILO/IPEC project on HIV-induced Child Labour in Sub-Saharan Africa (2004–2008), and ILO/IPEC project of Support to the National Action Plan on the Elimination of Child Labour in Uganda (2008–2012). Frank Hagemann, Head of Policy and Research, ILO/IPEC. Alice Ouedraogo, Deputy Director, ILO Policy Integration Department. Many other ILO/IPEC staff who, in one way or another, contributed to this article.

References

1 Towards Universal Access. UNAIDS Annual Report (2008) ISBN 978 92 9173 800. WHO, UNAIDS, UNICEF, Geneva

2 Uganda Bureau of Statistics, Uganda National Household Survey, (2006). Uganda Bureau of Statistics, Kampala.

3 Rau B (2006). The politics of civil society in confronting HIV/AIDS. *International Affairs* **82**(2):285–95.

4 Beauchemin E (1999). The exodus: The growing migration of children from Ghana's rural areas to the urban centres. Catholic Action for Street Children and UNICEF, Accra.

5 International Labour Organization (2003). Investing in every child: An economic study of the costs and benefits of eliminating child labour. ILO, Geneva.

6 ILO, IPEC (1997). Child labour in commercial agriculture in Africa, Report of Technical Workshop, Geneva.

7 Gabriel R (1999). HIV/AIDS and the commercial agricultural sector of Kenya, FAO/UNDP, Rome.

8 Kelly MJ (1999). The impact of HIV/AIDS on schooling in Zambia. Paper presented at the International Conference on AIDS and STDS in Africa, Lusaka.

9 Kelly, MJ (2001). Challenging the challenger, understanding and expanding the response of universities in Africa to HIV/AIDS. University of Zambia, Lusaka.

10 UNICEF (1999). Children orphaned by AIDS, front line responses from eastern and southern Africa. United Nations Children's Fund.

11 Foster G *et al.* (1995). Orphan prevalence and extended family care in a peri-urban community in Zimbabwe. *AIDS Care (London)*, **7**:3–17.

12 Tibajiuka A, Kaijage F (1995). Patterns and processes of social exclusion in Tanzania. In Rodgers GC *et al.* (eds), *Social Exclusion, Rhetoric, Reality, Responses*, pp. 187–200. Geneva/New York: ILO/UNDP.

13 Making a Difference for Children Affected By AIDS (2000). Population Council, Horizons Project Research Summary no. 3, Washington, DC. Available at http://www.popcouncil.org/horizons/ressum/orphans.html

14 UNAIDS (2000). Epidemiological fact sheet on HIV/AIDS and sexually transmitted infections for Zambia. Geneva

15 UNAIDS(2000). Report on the global HIV/AIDS epidemic. Geneva

16 ILO (2006). HIV/AIDS and work: Global estimates, impact on children and youth, and response. ILO, Geneva.

17 UNICEF, UNAIDS and USAID (2004). *Children on the brink 2004, A joint report of new orphans estimates and a framework for action.* July 2004, USAID, United Nations Childern's Fund, New York.

18 Out of the Shadows (2000). A worldwide report on the worst forms of child labour. Global March, New Delhi.

19 ILO/IPEC (2002). *Investigating the Worst Forms of Child Labour No.12: Children in Prostitution in Tanzania, A Rapid Assessment*, ILO, Geneva.

20 UNAIDS (2000). The impact of HIV/AIDS on developing countries. Social and Economic Development, International Development Committee, House of Commons, 18 July,United Kingdom.

21 International Labour Office (2001). *An ILO Code of Practice on HIV/AIDS and the world of work*, International Labour Organization, Geneva.

22 United Nations Commission on the Status of Women (2006), *Resolution on Women, the Girl Child and HIV/AIDS.* United Nations, New York.

23 ILO, *Plan of Action to combat HIV-induced child labour, ILO Tripartite Workshop on the Impact of HIV/AIDS on Child Labour in Sub-Saharan Africa.* ILO, Lusaka, 6–8. May 2003, available in: ILO/IPEC Project Combating and preventing HIV/AIDS-induced child labour in Sub-Saharan Africa: pilot action in Uganda and Zambia, ILO/IPEC Multi-bilateral Programme of Technical Cooperation 2004, Government of the United States of America, Governments of Uganda and Zambia (not published).

24 ILO/IPEC (2004), *Project Combating and preventing HIV/AIDS-induced child labour in Sub-Saharan Africa: pilot action in Uganda and Zambia*, ILO/IPEC Multi-bilateral Programme of Technical Cooperation, Government of the United States of America, Governments of Uganda and Zambia (not published).

25 Republic of Uganda, Ministry of Gender, Labour and Social Development, *National Child Labour Policy*, Ministry of Gender, Labour and Social Development, Kampala, November 2006.

26 World Bank (2000). Zimbabwe-multi-sectoral AIDS project Report no. PID9727. Washington, DC.

27 UNICEF, UNAIDS and USAID, *Children on the brink 2004, a joint report of new orphans estimates and a framework for action*, July 2004.

Chapter 9F

Illustrative example F: Psychosocial and developmental effects

Susan Gunn, David L. Parker, and Mary E. Miller

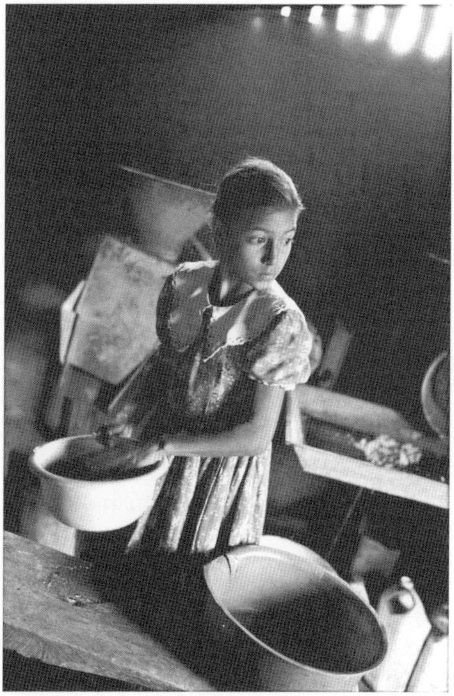

Domestic servant, Nicaragua

Introduction

Health – psychological as well as physical – is central to the definition of child labour in international law. The International Labour Organization (ILO) Conventions speak of the 'fullest physical and mental development of young persons' [1] and the United Nations Convention on the Rights of the Child declares that 'the child, by reason of his physical and mental immaturity, needs special safeguards and care, including appropriate legal protection' [2]. However, while the physical aspects of the working child's health are beginning to receive the attention they deserve, the non-physical aspects are not.

This chapter examines some of the issues surrounding child workers' psychological functioning and social/intellectual development (abbreviated as PSID) and considers how this important aspect of health might be better measured, monitored, and addressed.

The number of children affected by PSID risks is large. As of 2004, 126 million children aged 5–17 were estimated to be engaged in work which poses a health risk [3]. However, these estimates are based on physical risks only; the approximately 300 large-scale national surveys on which the most recent global statistics are based did not include PSID indicators. It is, therefore, likely that figures on children in hazardous work are underestimated and would rise once PSID is taken into account. In 2008 the ILO added a question on PSID[1] to its model questionnaire for national surveys which will be helpful in producing quantitative data in the future [4].

Research on PSID effects of children's work

Concern about PSID effects of child labour is not new. The issue was officially raised as early as 1972 in a special report of the World Health Organization (WHO), which noted that rapid technological changes, particularly mechanization in developing countries, were having an adverse effect on child workers' psychosocial health [5]. The 1984 meeting of the Joint ILO/WHO Committee on Occupational Health raised the issue again and instigated a series of descriptive studies of PSID factors associated with child work in four occupational sectors: domestic services [6], agriculture [7], street-based trades, and factory work. The latter was described as creating a great deal of stress for the child worker.

> Long hours and days of uninterrupted work have a stultifying effect on the child, narrowing his horizons and often crippling him emotionally. Since a child working full time with potentially dangerous machines cannot afford to imagine or fantasize, as most children do, the child's creativity and ability to transcend reality are blunted and his whole mental world becomes impoverished as a result [8].

Subsequently, several seminal works on child labour have urged that more consideration be given to PSID [9], but little primary research has ensued.

---

1 Have you ever been subject to the following at work?Constantly shouted atRepeatedly insultedBeaten/physically hurt...Sexually abused (touched or done things to you that you did not want)Other (Specify)

Instead, the PSID work which has been done has focused on the relatively small proportion of children engaged in armed conflict, trafficked, and/or exploited in sex-related occupations [10, 11, 12, 13].

However, as job stress has become increasingly recognized as a significant factor in adult occupational health in the US and Europe, some research has been undertaken on stress in young workers as well [14, 15]. Research into other conditions of work, although still very limited, indicate that work intensity (i.e. the number of work hours) and late night work by children have an impact on both their physical health, due to exhaustion and sleep deprivation, and on their psychosocial health [16, 17]. There is also a demonstrable effect of child labour on intellectual development.

Studies have shown that, with increased work hours, there is a decrease in school achievement, increased school drop-out rates, and disruption of family relationships [18]. An important area that is still not being researched at present is the psychosocial health impacts of injuries incurred during early work experience.

There is a growing number of specialized field studies in low and medium income countries on the impact of factors such as intimidation, isolation, violence, lack of stimulation, and harassment can have on children's psychosocial development. The following studies from Ethiopia, Bangladesh, Nepal, Jordan, Brazil, and the Philippines illustrate the point.

A study of public perceptions of child labour in Ethiopia found that beating, neglect and emotional abuse were viewed as the most frequently occurring types of abuse in child labour [19]. This finding led to an in-depth study of 1000 randomly selected children, aged 5–15, of whom 528 were domestics, street-workers, and private enterprise workers and 472 were controls. Over twice as many child labourers as controls exhibited anxiety disorders, and psychosocial stressors were one and half times more likely among the study subjects than in the control group [20].

A study was undertaken in Bangladesh of 4643 village children, aged 5–15, approximately 900 of whom were working over 4 hours a day. Twelve percent of the working children reported being beaten at work [21].

In a Jordanian study of 103 boys, aged 11–16 years working as mechanics, 61% reported physical abuse and 27% reported sexual abuse [22]. A study of 249 Nepalese child porters (aged 5–14 years) showed them to be at increased risk of sexual assault, general emotional distress, and early consumption of alcohol when compared to a group of 262 controls [23].

A cross-sectional study of 3139 children and adolescents from poor areas of the city of Pelotas in southern Brazil found that the risk of behavioural problems was 2.7 times greater among younger child workers when compared with adolescents and that behavioural problems were particularly associated with domestic service and starting work at an early age [24].

A Philippine study of child scavengers demonstrates the effect of work on intellectual development and how PSID findings can be used to address the identified deficits. A small sample of children aged 7–15 years was drawn from a health hazard study of 1200 scavenger children and a matched control group of non-working children from an adjoining slum. The children were evaluated using an extensive battery of psychosocial assessment tests especially validated for marginalized children (e.g. child prostitutes). While dexterity and social intelligence were shown to be similar for the two groups, the intellectual functioning of the child scavengers showed a progressive decline compared to the control group. The decline started at the age of 7 years with the difference becoming most marked in those aged 11–13 years. Noting that this latter age group was also the age when most child scavengers dropped out of school [25], several local public school teachers designed a special curriculum to strengthen the child scavengers' intellectual skills using visual and kinaesthetic modes of learning [26]. A follow-up study 10 years later demonstrated that the school completion rate was high among the child workers who participated in the programme [27].

Following a review of these and other health-related studies on child labour, Dorman concludes that: 'enough is known at this point to indicate that ... child labour could interfere with the process of psychological and social development' [28]. For those areas of PSID where research on child workers is still inadequate, other studies may be helpful, for example research on psychosocial health and development in non-working children, on children in difficult circumstances such as extreme poverty [29] and war [30], and on work-related psychosocial health of adults. Such studies can suggest lines of inquiry and identify ways of addressing the psychosocial conditions found, which is particularly important in the case of child workers.

Studies have also underscored the importance of factors, such as resilience, which serve to protect some children. Resilience is often linked to early support and close ties with family and peer group [31]. This and other potentially protective factors deserve much more attention. Although they do not negate psychosocial or developmental risks, they help mitigate their impact and facilitate development of intervention strategies.

The importance of incorporating PSID in legal instruments

Few countries of the world include reference to PSID in their child labour laws and regulations. The ILO Conventions on minimum age (No. 138) and on the worst forms of child labour (no. 182)[2] require countries to determine, i.e. to list, work which is likely to harm children's health, safety, or morals. The resulting lists of hazardous work are important because they serve as the basis for national legislation, local ordinances, and guidelines for labour inspectors, social workers, and many others. As such, they are an important indicator of what signatory countries formally recognize as dangerous work for children. While many work environments may cause or contribute to psychosocial harm, few governments have acknowledged this fact by listing a prohibited work environment or work activity based upon its likelihood to pose a psychosocial risk.

Figure 9F.1 presents data from a survey of 119 countries which illustrates what work the countries have listed.

As long as policy makers remain unaware of the importance of PSID problems resulting from work, these types of abusive conditions will continue to be excluded from hazardous child labour lists. The prime example is domestic service. It is probably the second most common form of child labour (after agriculture) and involves large numbers of girls. However, in 2005 only 14 countries listed domestic service or its associated tasks. This is in spite of the fact that in work environments where children are 'confined to the premises of the employer' and 'hidden work situations in which girls are at a special risk' is explicitly noted in Recommendation 190 accompanying ILO Convention no. 182 [33].

A framework for identifying and addressing PSID effects of child labour

The general lack of attention that has been given to PSID factors derives, in part, from the fact that methods traditionally used in PSID studies are ill-suited for work with large population groups and in the circumstances in which child labour generally occurs. Most of the existing tools for psychosocial evaluation tend to be expensive and are impractical for developing countries because the instruments require individual assessments and professional analyses. There are some notable exceptions: the general psychosocial framework developed by Martin Woodhead [34]; a detailed guide for labour inspectors and other field practitioners by Catherine Boidin [35]; a reference for use in rapid assessments by Judith Ennew [36]; and a special tool for assessing PSID in child domestic workers [37]. Currently, over 80 countries are conducting

[2] ILO Convention no. 182 has been ratified by 95% of all countries as of 2009. Ratification brings an obligation to undertake the actions outlined in the Convention, such as to prepare the list of hazardous work.

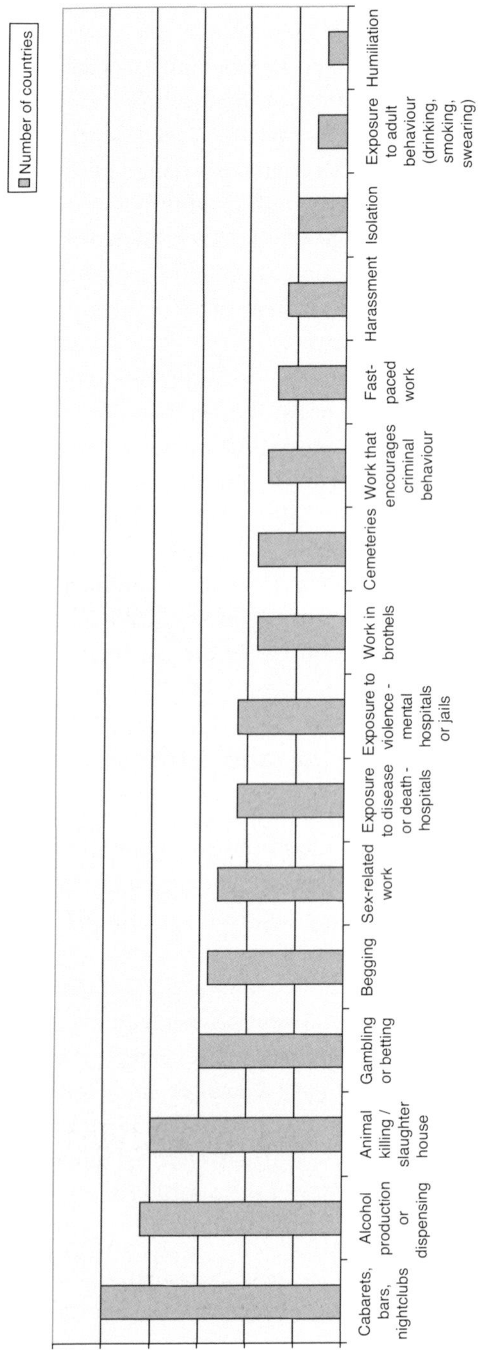

Fig. 9F.1 Types of work listed for prohibition due to psychosocial risk.
Source: ILO, 2005 [32]

child labour programmes, with target groups ranging in size from a few hundred to over 40,000. This work, as well as increasing concern worldwide for safe youth employment, has created a demand for methods that will enable the identification of PSID harm on a larger scale and facilitate the development of appropriate services to address this harm. Managers are requesting information on what constitutes both psychological and physical harm so they do not violate child labour laws with respect to adolescents aged 15–18 years. Assessment tools must be able to delineate the point at which work poses unacceptable risk.

As a first step to developing a tool with which to understand psychosocial stressors, it is useful to consider the different ways in which child labour can influence PSID. As seen in Table 9F.1, there are both positive and negative aspects to the impact of work. Building on a framework proposed by Woodhead, Table 9F.2 shows the major indicators of psychosocial function and development and the hazards which may compromise them.

Tools for examining these dimensions need to be simple to understand, easily validated, and readily administered [38]. Ideally, such tools would be standardized so that cross-cultural comparisons could be made; such comparisons would be an important means of understanding the overall dynamics and impacts of child labour [39].

The development of such tools could be accomplished by bringing together experts who can evaluate common developmental stages in children, regardless of their cultural background.

In the short term, countries of the European Union, India, and the US among others have tailored safety checklists for several trades in which young people commonly work. Incorporating PSID into occupational safety and health checklists is advantageous because they are used by labour inspectors and employers for identifying hazards, prioritizing them for action, and designing interventions. Other potential users of such comprehensive checklists could be social auditing firms which are overseeing supply chains for the international market, social welfare officers who assess families at risk, or even

Table 9F.1 Four dimensions of the psychosocial impact of work

	The work	The setting
Negatives	Psychosocial hazards due to the nature of the work (fast-paced, repetitive, excessive work hours or night shift)	Psychosocial hazards in the work environment (violence, exposure to adult habits, isolation)
Positives	Protective factors associated with the type of work (remuneration, learning opportunities)	Protective factors in the environment (working with others, policies against harassment, adequate supervision)

Table 9F.2 Psychosocial indicators and associated hazards

Psychosocial and development indicators	Examples of hazards which may impair function
Cognitive abilities and cultural competencies (e.g. intelligence, communication skills, technical skills)	Work involves monotonous and stultifying activities over long periods of time such as factory work or pounding stone into gravel
Personal security, social integration and social competence (e.g. secure attachments, positive adult/peer relations, social confidence, sense of belonging)	Breakdown of social networks; disruptions to familiar surroundings, isolation from peers and stigmatization as in domestic service
Personal identity and valuation (e.g. self-concept, self-esteem, feeling valued and respected)	Work in large groups producing low-value services or items as in quarries, or dumpsites
Sense of personal agency (e.g. self-efficacy, internal locus of control, positive outlook)	Situations where young workers, by virtue of their limited experience at work and in the labour market, have low job control
Emotional and somatic expressions of well-being (e.g. stress levels; sleeping and eating patterns, general health)	Situations where young worker are put at risk by carrying a heavy burden of responsibility for family and siblings

parents who must determine whether their children's work is appropriate. The use of well-crafted guidelines can also assist corporations in better defining the conditions under which children can work who are over the legal working age.

An alternative to the checklist approach is a system that enables early detection, documentation, and reporting of findings to the relevant authorities. Brazil has demonstrated that this is feasible on a large scale. The Ministry of Health commissioned guidelines, a database, and training materials, and then trained over 3500 front line health care providers (e.g. emergency room and hospital intake staff, personnel of rural and urban clinics) to recognize and to report work-related injuries, illnesses, and psychosocial problems among working children and young people. Initially the plan encountered considerable resistance as many health care workers considered it either unnecessary or beyond their capability [40]. However, once data started to demonstrate unexpected health conditions and that a significant number of children did have work-related health conditions, the programme was readily embedded in the health system.

Conclusions

The risks of various types of work to psychosocial functioning and intellectual development for children remain under-recognized and poorly researched, in large part because tested methods are not available for use with large population groups or under the conditions found in most developing countries. In many work situations, it is the PSID problems that will determine whether or not an occupation and/or work setting is harmful to children and therefore whether it is 'off-limits' to all those under age 18. Without means of diagnosing these conditions, action to address them will inevitably be insufficient. The importance of sensitizing policy makers, parents, employers, and the general public to psychological issues associated with child work cannot be underestimated. There are promising initiatives that demonstrate how this can be accomplished. However, a good evidence base is crucial. Since demonstrating the risks working children face from physical injury and exposures has been critical to protecting them, the widespread and serious psychosocial health effects must be given equivalent attention as well. As long as work-related harm continues to be considered within narrow physical parameters, large numbers of children will be left without adequate protection.

References

1 Article 1, ILO Minimum Age Convention, no. 138 (1973).

2 Preamble, Convention on the Rights of the Child (1989).

3 Hagemann F, Diallo Y, Etienne A, Mehran F (2006). *Global Child Labour Trends, 2000 to 2004*. Geneva: International Labour Organization.

4 International Labour Organization (2008). Available at http://www.ilo.org/ipec/ChildlabourstatisticsSIMPOC/Model%20questionnaires/lang–en/index.htm (accessed 21 October 2009).

5 World Health Organization (1987). Children at work: Special Health Risks. Report of a WHO Study Group, Geneva.

6 Onyango P and Kayongo-Male D (1982). *Psychological Effects of Child Labour*. Nairobi: University of Nairobi.

7 Taylor RB (1973). Sweatshops in the Sun: Child Labour on the Farm. Boston: Beacon Press.

8 Mendelievich E (1979). *Children at Work*. Geneva: International Labour Office.

9 Forssman S and Coppee GH (1973). Occupational health problems of young workers. Occupational Safety and Health Series, no. 26, International Labour Office, Geneva; Greenberger E and Steinberg L (1986). *When Teenagers work: The Psychological and Social Costs of Adolescent Employment*. New York: Basic Books; Forastieri V (1997). *Children at Work: Health and Safety Risks*. Geneva: International Labour Organization.

10 Zimmerman C, Hossain M, Yun K, Roche B, Morison L, and Watts C (2006). Stolen smiles: A summary report on the physical and psychological health consequences of women and adolescents trafficked in Europe, London School of Hygiene & Tropical Medicine, London.

11 Tanzania Media Women's Association (TAMWA) (2004). A report on the assessment of child sexual abuse and exploitation (unpublished paper) Dar es Salaam.

12 Betancourt TS and Khan KT (2008). The mental health of children affected by armed conflict: protective processes and pathways to resilience. *International Review of Psychiatry*;Betancourt TS and Williams T (2008). Building an evidence base on mental health interventions for children affected by armed conflict. War Trauma Foundation;Betancourt TS *et al.* 2008). Psychosocial adjustment and social reintegration of children associated with armed forces and armed groups: The state of the field and future directions. *Psychology Beyond Borders.* Available at http://psychologybeyondborders.com/Publications.aspx

13 Wessels M (2008). Do no harm: Challenges in organizing psychosocial support to displaced people in emergency settings. *Refuge*, **25**(1): 6–14.

14 National Research Council (1998). Protecting youth at work: Health, safety, and development of working children and adolescents in the United States. Washington, DC: National Academy Press, Institute of Medicine.

15 Copsey S (2009). Preventing risks to young workers: Policy, programmes and workplace practices. Luxembourg: European Agency for Safety and Health at Work, Working Environment Information.

16 Carskadon M (1990). Patterns of sleep and sleepiness in adolescents. *Pediatrician*, **17**:5–12.

17 Dornbusch SM (2004). Sleep and adolescence: A social psychologist's perspective. In Carskadon MA (ed.), *Adolescent Sleep Patterns: Biological, Social, and Psychological Influences*, pp. 1–3. Cambridge, UK: Cambridge University Press.

18 National Research Council (1998). Protecting youth at work: Health, safety, and development of working children and adolescents in the United States. Washington, DC: National Academy Press, Institute of Medicine.

19 Fekadu D and Alem A (2001). Child labour and emotional disorders in an urban district in Ethiopia: A rapid assessment on community perceptions of child labour (unpublished paper).

20 Fekadu D, Alem A, Hagglof B (2006). The prevalence of mental health problems in Ethiopian child laborers. *Journal of Child Psychology and Psychiatry*, **47**:954–9.

21 Hadi A (2000). Child abuse among working children in rural Bangladesh: Prevalence and determinants. *Public Health*, **114**:380–4 (quoted in Dorman (2008). Child *Labour Education and Health: A Review of the Literature, Understanding Child Work.* Geneva: World Bank, ILO, UNICEF.

22 Gharaibeh M and Hoeman S (2003). Health hazards and risks for abuse among child labor in Jordan. *Journal of Pediatric Nursing*, **18**(2):140–7.

23 Doocy S, Crawford B, Boudreaux C, Walla E, (2007). The risks and impacts of portering on the well-being of children in Nepal. *Journal of Tropical Pediatrics*, **53**: 165–70.

24 Benvegnu LA, Fassa AG, Facchini LA, Wegman DH, Dall'Agnol MM (2005). Work and behavioural problems in children and adolescents. *International Journal of Epidemiology* **34**(6):1417–24.

25 Torres EB, Subida RD, Rabuco LB (1991). The profile of child scavengers in Smokey Mountain, Balut, Tondo, Manila. University of Philippines, College of Public Health Working Paper, Manila.

26 Gunn S, Ostos Z (1992). Dilemmas in tackling child labour: The case of scavenger children in the Philippines. *International Labour Review*, **131**(6):

27 Salamat A (2003). Smokey Mountain project: Follow-up Study (unpublished evaluation), International Labour Organization, Manila.

28 Dorman P (2008). *Child Labour Education and Health: A Review of the Literature, Understanding Child Work*, p.44. Geneva: World Bank, ILO, UNICEF.

29 Dawes A, Donald D (2000). *Child-Context Relationships and Developmental Outcomes: Some Perspectives on Poverty and Culture.* Richmond, Virginia: Christian Children's Fund.

30 Catani C, Schauer E, Elbert T, Missmahl I, Bette JP, Neuner F (2009). War trauma, child labor, and family violence: Life adversities and PTSD in a sample of school children in Kabul. *Journal of Trauma and Stress*, **22**(3):163–71.

31 Caffo E, Belaise C (2003). Psychological aspects of traumatic injury in children and adolescents. *Child and Adolescent Psychiatric Clinics of North America*, 12(3):493–535.

32 International Programme on the Elimination of Child Labour (2005). *Steps Toward Determining Hazardous Child Labour: A Toolkit of Reference Materials and Practical Examples.* Geneva: ILO.

33 ILO Recommendation 190 (1999). Paragraph 3(e) and paragraph 2(c)iii accompanying ILO Convention on the worst forms of child labour no.182.

34 Woodhead M (2004). *Psychosocial Impacts of Child Work: Research, Monitoring, and Intervention, Understanding Child Work series.* New York: World Bank, ILO, UNICEF.

35 Boidin C (1995). Labour inspection and the adoption of a policy on child labour. The working child: Psychosociological approach. Labour Administration Branch Document no. 42, International Labour Office, Geneva.

36 Ennew J (1994). Rapid assessment procedure (RAP) for the field of child labour: Psycho-social measurement of hazards of work or working conditions. ILO Unpublished Report, Geneva.

37 Brewer SE (2005). Tool for assessing the psychological effects of child domestic work. An Anti-Slavery International Working Document, London.

38 LaMontagne AD, Keegel T, Vallance D (2007). Protecting and promoting mental health in the workplace: Developing a systems approach to job stress. *Health Promotion Journal of Australia*, **18**(3):221–8.

39 Woodhead M (2009). Harmed by work or developing through work? Issues in the study of psychosocial impacts. Unpublished Manuscript).

40 Barker, SL (2008). How to include the health sector in the public policies for the eradication of child labour: The Brazilian experience. ILO- IPEC Working Paper, Geneva.

Part 3

The global response to child labour and its impact: Case studies

Chapter 10

Country-wide case studies: Brazil – A focus on conditional cash transfers

Ana Lúcia Kassouf

Introduction

Human capital plays an important role in the process of economic growth and development. At a micro-level, schooling years is related to capacity and productivity and consequently higher earnings and better jobs. Poor health can affect an individual's opportunities, such as earning capacity, school performance, ability to care for children, and participation in community activities. Similarly, education is an important determinant of an individual's income, health, and capacity to interact and communicate with others.

Conditional cash transfer (CCT) programmes have become widespread in some less economically developed countries. Their purpose is to alleviate poverty and invest in human capital. Poor families receive money from governments as a complementary income source tied to certain conditions such as visiting health facilities, immunizing children, and enrolling children in school. The cash transfers aim to cover the direct costs of schooling (e.g. school fees, books, uniforms), and the indirect opportunity cost of time not spent in school, for example a reduction in the time children spend working. The two largest conditional cash transfer programmes are Mexico's *Oportunidades* and Brazil's *Bolsa Família.*

This chapter is the first of three county-wide case studies examining the impact of national policies to tackle child labour. These policies are examined in the context of the public health model of child labour discussed throughout this book. In the context of Brazil this chapter examines in particular the *Bolsa Escola* and *Bolsa Família* programmes, and the *Child Labour Eradication Programme*. In terms of the model of child labour discussed throughout this book, in Brazil it has been principally on legislative, educational, and economic measures.

Child labour in Brazil

The 2007 Brazilian National Household Survey reported that the number of working children aged 5–15 years exceeded 2.5 million or 6.6% of all children in this age group. A further 2.3 million or 35% of adolescents aged 16–17 years worked. Of these 38% worked in agriculture and livestock activities, 21% are in service, 20% in commerce, 12% in the industry sector, and 5% in civil construction. Most young women and girls worked in services, such as domestic work, while males were more likely to work in the agricultural sector [1].

During the last two decades, there has been a large decrease in the proportion of children and adolescents working in Brazil. This fall in child labour, along with the increase in school attendance has been accompanied by improving socioeconomic conditions.

National policy measures to address child labour in Brazil

Policy and legislative change

The Brazilian Constitutions of 1934, 1937, and 1946 set and confirmed a minimum working age of 14 years. In 1967, however, during the military dictatorship, the minimum working age was lowered to 12 years. This was again revised in the 1988 Constitution, which prohibited any form of night and hazardous work in children aged less than 18 years of age, and any other form of labour in children under the age of 14 years, with the exception of professional training and apprenticeship programmes. A constitutional amendment passed in December 1998 increased the minimum age to 16 years except for apprentices, in which case the minimum age is 14 years.

During the 1990s, the Federal Government instituted major policy changes. The minimum working age was increased to 16 years. The implementation of a National Education Law established minimum levels of spending per child in school, decentralized school decision-making authority and set minimum teacher training levels [2]. A special fund was established to increase school funding, especially for poor regions of the country [3].

At the same time as these latter legislative changes, a media campaign with input from international organizations, such as ILO and UNICEF was undertaken to raise awareness and promote action to stop the exploitation of children.

Direct support: The Bolsa Escola and Bolsa Família Programmes

The contribution of children's earnings to household income is important, mainly because in the households where there are working children, the per capita income is very low. This is explored more fully in the economics section of this book. In 31% of households the contribution of children's earnings to the household's income is more than 20% and in almost 9% of the households the contribution of children's earnings to the household income is more than 40% [4]. In families in which children's contribution to household income is high, social programmes are very important. The grants paid to poor families have the potential therefore to stop children working and to see them enrolled in school.

The Conditional Cash Transfer Programme started in 1995 in Brazil in the cities of Brasilia (also called the Federal District) and Campinas (located in São Paulo state). The programme provided a stipend (cash payments) to poor families with children from 7 to 14 years old conditional on their children being enrolled in school and attending at least 85% of school days. By 1998, more than 50 *municípios* in 7 of the 26 states of Brazil (plus the Federal District) had adopted a similar programme.

In April 2001, the Federal *Bolsa Escola* Programme was created under President Fernando Henrique Cardoso. According to the Social and Development Ministry by the end of 2001, almost 5 million families with children from 6 to 15 years old were receiving a stipend in more than 5000 out of a total of 5560 *municípios*. In 2003, under President Luis Inacio Lula da Silva, *Bolsa Escola* became *Bolsa Família*, and the programme's benefits were expanded.

By 2006 the government budget for *Bolsa Família* had reached more than 7.5 billion Reais (about 4 billion US dollars), representing 0.35% of GNP. And by 2007, according to the Ministry of Social Development, more than 11 million families, or about 46 million people (about one-fourth of Brazil's population) were beneficiaries of the programme. The number of beneficiaries was larger in urban areas (5.5 million families receiving *Bolsa Família*) compared to rural areas (2.6 million families receiving *Bolsa Família*). However, 31.3% of the households in rural areas were receiving stipends, while in urban areas the percentage was 11.9% [4].

While *Bolsa Escola* included only poor families with children from 6 to 15 years old, *Bolsa Família* included all families with monthly per capita incomes below 60.00 Reais (30.00 dollars) and families with monthly per capita incomes between 60.00 and 120.00 Reais that also had children from newborn to 15 years old or a pregnant or breastfeeding woman. The *Bolsa Família* programme was expanded in March 2008 to include 16- and 17-year-old youth. The stipends provided by *Bolsa Família* are usually paid to a woman in the household, either the head or the wife, through a bank card. This is done because studies have shown that women are better at managing financial resources in a way that improves the well-being of their families [5, 6, 7].

The monthly stipend paid to families ranges from 20 Reais (approximately US$ 10) to 182 Reais (approximately US$ 90), depending on the family's income and number of children.

Conditional cash transfer programmes are often preferred to standard income transfer programmes because of the conditions they impose on families. For example, the *Bolsa Família* requires that each child between the ages of 6 and 17 years be enrolled in school and attend at least 85% of school days, that pregnant women obtain prenatal and postnatal health care services and those between newborn and 7 years of age receive their recommended vaccinations. The increase in human capital that should result from increased education and better health status is intended to allow families to break out of their cycle of poverty, improve their quality of life and end their dependence on public assistance.

The Child Labour Eradication Programme

In 1996 the Federal Government launched the *Child Labour Eradication Programme* with the specific goal of eradicating child labour. It started in selected states, and focused on children living in rural areas and engaged in dangerous activities. Later on the programme was expanded nationwide to urban areas. This programme provided monthly cash payments to families with children between the age of 7 and 14 and with a per capita income below half the minimum monthly wage. The conditions are an agreement to withdraw the child from work and to maintain them attending regular school and after-school programme, called *Jornada Ampliada*. In Brazil, children typically have a four or five hour day in school. Thus the after-school program should support families that have difficulties in taking care of children while they are not at school as well as providing sports, culture, artistic, and leisure opportunities.

The programme also aims to promote the social inclusion of families through adult participation in socio-educative activities and in projects of professional qualification and thereby to generate employment and income. According to the Ministry of Social Development, in 2005, one million children were beneficiaries of the *Child Labour Eradication Programme*, with the government budget reaching 220 million US dollars. In 2005, the *Child Labour Eradication Programme* was integrated with the *Bolsa Família* with the added condition that there should be no working children in beneficiary families.

The impact of national policy measures to address child labour in Brazil

Most of the research that has taken place on the impact of efforts to reduce child labour in Brazil has focused on the conditional cash transfer programmes.

The best evidence for the impact of conditional cash transfer programmes actually comes from Mexico where the *Progresa* programme was implemented in a randomized fashion creating the research conditions for a more robust evaluation [8, 9, 10, 11, 12, 13]. This is discussed more fully in the education section of this book. There has also been some research from Bangladesh on the *Food for Education* programme [14]. Probably reflecting the more extensive research that has taken place on Mexico's *Progresa* programme, only a few studies have evaluated the impact of Brazil's *Bolsa Escola* and *Bolsa Família* programmes.

Bourguignon *et al.* analysed Brazilian household survey data collected in 1999 to construct a model of household behaviour that was used to simulate the future impact of the *Bolsa Escola* programme [15]. They estimated that the programme would result in more than half of the eligible youths who were not in school enrolling in school, but that there would be no effect on child labour. It should be noted that this paper was an economic exercise, and it should not now be interpreted as an assessment of the actual impact of the *Bolsa Escola* and *Bolsa Família* programmes.

Other papers have sought to estimate the actual impact of Brazilian conditional cash transfer programme on children's and parents' labour status and on children's school enrolment. For example, Cardoso and Souza and Ferro and Kassouf both concluded that the *Bolsa Escola* and *Bolsa Família* programmes have had a large positive impact on school enrolment [16, 17]. Although they had no effect in reducing child labour participation, the actual number of hours worked by children decreased. These studies, however, used cross-sectional data from 2000 and 2001 and did little to control for selection into the programme. Ferro *et al.* using household survey data from 2003, however, showed that the programme reduced children's participation in work [18].

The majority of studies evaluating the impact of Brazil's *Bolsa Escola* and *Bolsa Familia* programmes have analysed data from the late 1990s and early 2000s. Since then the *Bolsa* programme has become widespread nationally and there is now a need for new research to analyse the impact of the programme given that several years have passed.

A more recent and thorough study was undertaken by Glewwe and Kassouf in 2008 [19]. This study used school-census data of eight years from 1998 to 2005. The study compared changes in school enrolment and school dropout, and grade advancement rates across schools that adopted the *Bolsa* programme at different times. The authors estimated that, after accounting for cumulative effects, the Bolsa program has increased enrolment in Brazil by about 5.5% in grades 1–4 and by about 6.5% in grades 5–8. They also estimate that the programme has lowered dropout rates by about 0.5 percentage points and raised grade promotion rates by about 0.9 percentage points for children in grades 1–4, and has reduced dropout rates by about 0.4 percentage points and increased grade promotion rates by about 0.3 percentage points for children in grades 5–8. Only about one-third of Brazil's children participate in the *Bolsa* programme, so the assumption that these results are due only to the impact of the programme on participants, with no effect on non-participants, implies that the impact of participating in the *Bolsa* programme is about three times higher than these estimates. Therefore, the long-run effect of the programme appears to be to increase participants' enrolment rates by about 18%, to reduce dropout rates by 1.5% and to raise grade promotion rates by 2%.

Research on the *Child Labour Eradication Programme* has been less extensive. Using data from children in municipalities that had implemented the *Child Labour Eradication Programme* in three states of the north-eastern region of Brazil (Bahia, Pernambuco, and Sergipe) and using the principles of an experimental design, Yap *et al.* found an increase in time spent in school, a decrease in child labour time and in risky work, and improvements in school measured by grade-for-age for those participating in the programme [20]. These findings were in contrast to the non-participant children who were found to work longer hours after the implementation of *Child Labour Eradication Programme.*

Sedlacek and Gustafsson-Wright analysed a social assessment on the *Child Labour Eradication Programme* and concluded that "families were satisfied with the *Jornada Ampliada's* ability to provide stimulus for their children and to provide a nutritional supplement". However, they noted that there was a lack of a curriculum based on a clear pedagogical strategy [21].

Conclusions

Human capital is associated with the well-being of society. Education and health affect the capacity of individuals to engage in economic, social, and political life. Inequalities in education, health, and income translate into inequalities in opportunity and are often accompanied by differences in power, influence, and social status. According to the 2006 World Development Report 'greater equity can reduce poverty, enhance economic growth, advance development, and deliver increased opportunities to the poorest groups in our societies' [22].

It is important to keep in mind the close interaction between education, health, and income. Well-educated parents invest more in their children's education and health. As child health increases, measured by height-for-age, the probability of being enrolled in school increases. Better nourished children have higher cognitive abilities and perform better in school. Individuals with more human capital and better risk management capabilities are able to reduce income oscillation and increase their well-being. These findings are not exclusive to Brazil [23, 24, 25]. Other studies show improvements in cognitive development and school performance as iron is supplemented to anaemic children, while studies on intestinal parasites have shown that drug treatment improves cognitive and education outcomes [26, 27].

Conditional cash transfer programmes play a potentially important role therefore not just in providing benefits to poor families but also at the same time, in improving the educational level and the health status of children and other family members and thereby improving their quality of life both in the short and long term. Parents will consider transferring their children from work to full time education not only if school and education of sufficient quality is available, but also if they are able to overcome the economic barriers to have their children enrol in school. This includes the direct cost of schooling such as books and uniforms, as well as the opportunity cost – the value of the work children might have to give up if they increase their school participation.

It is perhaps not surprising that given the size of the *Bolsa Família* programme; it benefits more than 11 million families, there have been problems reported both in the media and in academic studies. The main reported problems have been a perception that it creates welfare dependency, client fraud, errors of the exclusion of the poor and inclusion of the non-poor, duplicated benefits, and that there is a lack of monitoring of the programme.

The *Bolsa Família* programme has been criticized because it does not take account of the increase in the opportunity cost of time as a child gets older, and also because it does not take into account regional differences. The same amount of money is provided for primary school level children as to high school children and to families living in the Southeast, which is a relatively rich region, as in the Northeast, which is a poor region in Brazil. Moreover, routine labour inspection to gauge its effects on decrease child labour is almost non-existent in the informal sector and rural areas, where most child work takes place.

Most evaluations of the conditional cash transfer programme in Brazil, however, have been positive and show a decrease in poverty, income inequality as well as a decrease in child labour, and an increase in health and educational outcomes. Better monitoring of how the programme affects child labour and school enrolment is, however, essential if the programme is to be effective in its aim to increase families' human capital and to break the cycle of poverty.

References

1 Brazilian National Household (2007). PNAD. Pesquisa Nacional por Amostra de Domicílios (National Household Survey). IBGE, Rio de Janeiro.

2 LDB (1996). Lei de Diretrizes e Bases da Educação Nacional. Ministério da Educação. http://portal.mec.gov.br/arquivos/pdf/ldb.pdf

3 FUNDEF (1996). Fundo de Manutenção e Desenvolvimento do Ensino Fundamental e de Valorização do Magistério. Ministério da Educação. http://www.conselhos.mg.gov.br/uploads/15/file/quadrocomparativofundebfundef.pdf

4 Brazilian National Household Survey, (2004). PNAD. Pesquisa Nacional por Amostra de Domicílios (National Household Survey). IBGE, Rio de Janeiro.

5 Kassouf AL, Senauer B (1996). Direct and indirect effects of parental education on malnutrition among children in Brazil: A full income approach. *Economic Development and Cultural Change*, **44**(4):817–38.

6 Thomas D (1997). Incomes, expenditures, and health outcomes: Evidence on intra-household resource allocation. In Haddad L, Hoddinott J, Alderman H (eds), *Intrahousehold Resource Allocation in Developing Countries: Methods, Models, and Policy.* Baltimore, MD: The Johns Hopkins University Press.

7 Smith LC, Ramakrishnan U, Ndiaye A, Haddad L, Martorell R (2003). The Importance of women's status for child nutrition in developing countries. IFPRI, Research Report no. 131. Available at http://www.ifpri.org/pubs/ABSTRACT/abstr131.htm.

8 Schultz TP (2000). The impact of Progresa on school enrolments. International Food Policy Research Institute, Washington, DC.

9 Schultz TP (2004). School subsidies for the poor: Evaluating the Mexican PROGRESA poverty program. *Journal of Development Economics*, **74**:199–250.

10 Parker S, Rubalcava L, Teruel G (2008). Evaluating Conditional Schooling and Health Programs. In Schultz TP, Strauss J (eds), *Handbook of Development Economics*, Vol. 4. Amsterdam: Elsevier.

11 Behrman J, Sengupta P, Todd P (2000). The impact of PROGRESA on achievement test scores in the first year. International Food Policy Research Institute, Washington, DC.

12 Dubois P, de Janvry A, Sadoulet E (2004). Effects on school enrollment and performance of a conditional tranfers program in México. Department of Agricultural & Resource Economics, University of California, Berkeley.

13 Skoufias E, Parker S (2001). Conditional cash transfers and their impact on child work and schooling: Evidence from the PROGRESA program in Mexico. FCND Discussion Paper no. 123. International Food Policy Research Institute, Washington, DC.

14 Ravallion M, Wodon Q (2000). Does child labor displace schooling? Evidence on behavioral responses to an enrollment subsidy. *Economic Journal*, **110**, c158–75.

15 Bourguignon F, Ferreira F, Leite P (2003). Conditional cash transfers, schooling and child labor: Micro-simulating Brazil's *Bolsa* Escola Program. *World Bank Economic Review*, **17**(2):229–54.

16 Cardoso E, Souza AP (2003). The impact of income transfers on child labor and school attendance in Brazil. São Paulo: USP. Available at http://www.econ.fea.usp.br/elianacardoso/ ECONBRAS/cardoso-souza.pdf.

17 Ferro AR, Kassouf AL (2005). Avaliação do impacto dos programas *Bolsa* Escola sobre o trabalho infantil no Brasil. *Pesquisa e Planejamento Econômico*, **35**:417.

18 Ferro AR, Kassouf AL, Levison D (2007). The impact of conditional cash transfer program in Brazil on household work decisions in Brazil. Research in Labor Economics. Editors: S. Polachek and K. Tatsiramos. Emerald Press, Bingley, UK. (forthcoming).

19 Glewwe P, Kassouf AL (2008). The Impact of the Bolsa Escola/Familia Conditional Cash Transfer Program on Enrollment, Drop Out Rates and Grade Promotion in Brazil. (mimeo).

20 Yap YT, Sedlacek G, Orazem PF (2001). Limiting child labour through income transfers: An experimental evaluation of the PETI programme in rural Brazil, Inter-American Development Bank, Washington, DC (mimeo).

21 Sedlacek G and Wright G (2001). Eradicating child labor in Brazil. Report no. 21858-BR. Human Development Department, World Bank.

22 World Development Report (2006). *Equity and development.* Oxford University Press: World Bank.

23 Glewwe P, Jacoby H (1995). An economic analysis of delayed primary school enrollment in a low income country: The role of early childhood nutrition. *Review of Economic Statistics*, **77**(1):156–69.

24 Alderman H, Behrman J, Lavy V, Menon R (2001). Child health and school enrollment. *Journal of Human Resources*, **36**(1):185–205.

25 Glewwe P, Miguel EA (2008). The impact of child health and nutrition on education in less developed countries. *Handbook of Development Economics*, vol. 4. Amsterdam: Elsevier.

26 Nokes C, Van den Bosh C, Bandy D (1998). The effects of iron deficiency and anemia on mental and motor performance, educational achievement, and behavior in children: A report of the international nutritional anemia consultative group. Washington, DC: USAID.

27 Kvalsig JD, Cooppan RM, Connolly KJ (1991). The effects of parasite infections on cognitive processes in children. *Annals of Tropical Medicine and Parasitology*, **73**:501–6.

Chapter 11

Country-wide case studies: Kenya – A focus on ILO/IPEC and the Time Bound Programme

Philista Onyango

Introduction

Child labour has existed in Kenya since the colonial era. In the past, efforts were made to address it through initiatives led by charismatic individuals such as Bishop Owen. Following independence in 1963, the political leadership was more inclined to deny its existence. A cross-sectional study of child labour was undertaken by researchers from the University of Nairobi between 1982 and 1985 [1] and updated by the International Labour Organization (ILO) in 1991. In both studies, it was apparent that child labour was widespread in Kenya, in particular, in agriculture and in domestic service. This paved the way for an introduction of ILO/IPEC programmes in the country in 1992.

Many important factors contribute to child labour in Kenya. These include: poverty, particularly in rural areas and in informal urban settlements; an HIV/AIDS pandemic, which has left some 1.1 million children without parents; insecurity and conflict as witnessed in the 2008 post-election violence; domestic violence, longstanding social values and practices, such as sending children to herd cattle, to stay with relatives or to be married at an early age; and weak public institutions which hinder the implementation of policies and the enforcement of labour laws. Other factors contributing to child labour include; an informal and unregulated market that exists on low wages and does not attract adult labour; and the large number of vulnerable children who are forced by unscrupulous individuals to break into houses or traffic illicit goods across borders [2, 3, 4].

This chapter is one of three country-wide case studies examining the impact of national policies to tackle child labour. With regard to Kenya, this chapter examines two programmes introduced by ILO in 1992 and 2004 known as the ILO/IPEC Country Programme and Time Bound Programme. The focus in Kenya has been principally on raising awareness to change attitudes and practices and policy, on legislative reforms to enhance implementation and enforcement, and on direct support to enable children to attend school and acquire skills.

Child labour in Kenya

According to a 1998–1999 Central Bureau of Statistics (CBS) study, 1.9 million children aged 5–17 years were working in Kenya of whom 51.8% were boys and 48.2% girls. Most children were engaged in agriculture (56%) or domestic service (17%) [2]. In 2005–2006, the Kenyan Integrated Household Budget Survey reported that the number or working children had fallen to just over 950,000: a reduction of almost 1 million [5]. The Kenyan Integrated Household Budget Survey study found 773,696 actual child labourers, of whom 34% were working and attending school and 66% were not attending school [6]. Neither survey included street children whose numbers have been estimated at 700,000 [4].

More recent studies have confirmed that many children continue to work across a range of sectors including; street work such as hawking, vending and begging, mining, quarrying, construction, trafficking and transporting illicit and legal goods, and commercial sex work [7, 8, 9]. The introduction of free primary education in 2003 has reduced child labour and even the number of children seen on the streets, although this has still to be ascertained [10].

National policy measures and programmes to address child labour in Kenya

The Programmes

In 1992, Kenya was the first beneficiary of an ILO/IPEC Country-wide Programme in an agreement between the Ministry of Labour and the ILO. This included financial assistance for 10 years. To implement the programme, a multi-sectoral committee called the National Steering Committee on Child Labour was constituted. Led by the Ministry of Labour and Human Resource Development, the committee comprised employers, workers organizations, ministries, and non-governmental organizations (NGOs) working in children's sector.

At the introduction of the programme, many children were out of school due to poverty, and many families could not afford the school fees and other school levies that had been introduced as part of structural adjustment policies. There was no national child labour policy and legislation on child protection was weak. Child labour awareness levels were low and the relevant public and non-governmental institutions were virtually non-existent. The ILO/IPEC Programme focused on four broad areas: policy development and legislative reform; capacity building for policy implementation and law enforcement; awareness raising and social mobilization; and direct support to withdraw children from work and protect those at risk of dropping out of school. The overall Programme had 73 specific action programmes that were to be implemented by 25 organizations [11].

Policy and legislative measures

At the start of the ILO/IPEC Programme, there was no child labour policy and relevant legislation was through various unconnected statutes making it difficult to implement. Despite ratification of ILO Convention 138 on the Minimum Age for Employment and the UN Convention on the Rights of the Child, these two important documents had not been incorporated into domestic law.

Several studies on child labour were undertaken with the support of IPEC and the findings were widely disseminated through the media, conferences, seminars, and workshops to a range of stakeholders that included civil society groups, employers' and workers' representatives, government ministries and departments, teachers, children, and the public at large. The result of the consultation was a recommendation that a child labour policy be introduced and the Employment Act be overhauled.

A national policy on child labour was then formulated, a new Employment Bill drafted and the 2001 Children's Act enacted. Education was explicitly stated as crucial for tackling child labour. For example, under the Children's Act of 2001, child labour is clearly defined, and every child in Kenya is entitled to free and compulsory basic education. In addition, every child is protected from economic exploitation and any work that is likely to be hazardous or interfere with the child's education or harmful to a child's health or physical, mental, spiritual, moral, or social development [12].

With the new Children's Act in place, the government embarked on a review of the Education Act and formulated a new education policy. Again, recognizing that accessible, quality education was vital in tackling child labour; the policy provided for free primary education. This was followed with the development of an Education Sector Support Programme for 2005–2010. This programme set out measurable goals and targets for the implementation of the policy.

A new Employment Act, enacted in 2007, incorporated ILO Conventions 138 and 182. The Act defined child labour as it was in the Children's Act of 2001 and banned the worst forms of child labour. It also prohibited the employment of children less than13 years of age in any setting. If properly enforced, the Employment Act would increase children's participation in education and increase skills training. This has been a problem in Kenya, especially for those leaving school after just 8 years of education [13].

The National Plan of Action on Elimination of Child Labour

In order to implement the policy on child labour and to conform with ILO Convention 182 on Worst Forms of Child Labour, the government developed a National Plan of Action (National Plan). The National Plan's goal was to eliminate child labour with a focus on the worst forms [14]. Although the National Plan was supposed to be funded by the government, the Time Bound Programme funded its activities for 4 years.

Implementation of the National Plan was led by an Inter-Ministerial Coordinating Committee chaired by the Office of Vice President, assisted by a National Steering Committee composed of key government departments, Workers' and Employers' Unions, NGOs, and Faith-Based Organizations. At the ministerial level, the Division of Child Labour was to coordinate implementation activities, mainstream child labour into other government programmes and provide a secretariat to the National Steering Committee and the Inter-Ministerial Coordination Committee.

The National Plan outlined various actions. These included: prevention to ensure that children did not start working and those who were removed did not return to hazardous employment; protection of children who had to work by ensuring a safe environment free from hazardous work; prosecution of those found to be breaking the law; and partnership with statutory and non-governmental organizations. The target groups for National Plan were children working in agriculture, domestic service; commercial sex; street work, mines and quarries; construction and in the transport sector.

At district level the National Plan was implemented through the already established district and local child labour committees, and where there were none, new ones were to be created. The funding of the National Plan was to come from the government of Kenya.

The National Plan linked its activities with national social and economic development plans for Kenya and thereby addressed some of the root causes of child labour, such as poverty, unemployment and inequity. Under the National Plan, by 2012 net enrolment in education and training was to have increased to 95% while transition rates to technical institutions and universities were to have increased to 8 and 3%, respectively. Disadvantaged and marginalized groups were to be targeted with improved access to business opportunities, health, and education services. The plan was to reduce inequity by targeting development funds at poor families and communities.

In 2003, in addition to primary education, the government introduced bursary funds targeting poor families whose children were starting secondary schools. Constituency Development Funds were identified for meeting school levies, building classrooms, and buying books and desks. Given the large number of orphans, especially those related to AIDS, a Cash Transfer Fund (a form of conditional cash transfer) supporting families taking care of orphans was introduced. A bi-monthly stipend of KShs.3000 (US$38) was distributed to families taking care of an orphan on condition that the child attended school if of school age, was immunized, fed, had a birth registration, and had health records kept by the guardian.

Education, training and direct support through the Time Bound Programme

Children at risk of dropping out of school were identified and supported. Measures were taken to withdraw children from worst forms of child labour and return them either to school if they were aged less than 15 years or send them for skills training if they were aged 15 years or more. Certain schools were targeted with funds for income-generating activities as a means of sustaining the project once IPEC funding ended. The Time Bound Programme also supported efforts towards implementing free primary education. The families of withdrawn children were given funds to engage in income-generating activities, and assisted with accessing micro credit schemes and other financial supporting programmes in their communities.

Awareness raising, addressing values, and social mobilization

Most Kenyans were unaware of the hazardous working conditions faced by many children. Changing attitudes was identified as a priority area and different strategies including media and the arts were used to raise awareness among different groups ranging from policy makers to local communities.

Research, monitoring, and establishing a knowledge base

At the start of the ILO-IPEC Programme, accurate research and monitoring information on child labour was scanty. A child labour survey was conducted through the Integrated Labour Force Survey in 1998–1999. This was the first comprehensive source of data on child labour and was followed by sector-based baseline studies on child labour conducted by universities and other research institutions [5].

The Kenya National Bureau of Statistics through its routine labour force surveys incorporated a child labour module in the Integrated Household Budget Survey of 2005–2006 to update data on the labour force, which included labour of children. Surveys included children as young as 5 years.

The impact of national child labour policy measures and programmes in Kenya

Capacity building – Leadership and ownership

The arrival of ILO/IPEC Country Programme found Kenya implementing World Bank Structural Adjustment Policies. As a result of these policies Kenya was economically challenged, many children had dropped out of school, child labour was not considered a major issue, and there was little political support to address it. The first challenge was therefore to integrate the Country-wide Programme within the Kenyan context.

Although the National Steering Committee was supposed to coordinate the implementation of the ILO/IPEC Programme, the implementation role was in effect taken over by ILO/IPEC. The formal evaluation report stated that most of the institutional structures remained dysfunctional: the National Steering Committee hardly met; the Division of Child Labour within the Ministry of Labour remained understaffed; and child labour committees, which were seen as viable structures to monitor child labour at community level, did not work as their members had other responsibilities and their child labour role was not explicit in their official job description or performance contract [11]. The ILO/IPEC then took on the major role and the government role was minimal with a resultant failure to build national and local capacity, capability, and leadership in child labour. Thus, the fight against child labour by and large remained ILO/IPEC's responsibility. This limited the success of the programme. The final evaluation of the programme has not recorded any change and the verdict is the same: namely that the government has not owned the programme [20].

Policy and legislative change

The development of a national policy and a National Programme of Action on child labour was a major achievement and provided a framework for combating child labour and eliminating the worst forms [15]. The National Plan was ambitious at strategic and operational level. There was to be leadership and integration at the highest levels in government, and widespread dissemination down to district and community level. Major and longstanding health, social, educational, and economic inequalities in the country were to be reversed through poverty reduction programmes. Specific, newly-created funds created would help redistribute wealth.

The envisaged level of leadership did not materialize and there were problems with national funding commitments, however, new bursaries and development funds were introduced. A large part of these funds have been used in education by constructing classrooms to accommodate more children, buy books and desks for children, and thus facilitated the implementation of the free primary education policy.

Both the new 2001 Children's Act [12] and 2007 Employment Act [13] clearly and consistently defined child labour and made provisions regarding children's employment. The age at which a child enters light work has been reduced from 16 to 14 years to harmonize it with the age at which children in Kenya complete primary education. Both Acts have provisions on worst forms of child labour and on the right to compulsory basic education (from nursery to secondary education). The government has developed a policy on pre-school education and started subsidizing secondary education with the aim of attaining free basic education by 2015 [16].

The Time Bound Programme has produced some concrete results. These include; improved capacity and capability of newly formed institutions and partnerships, the establishment of a hazardous child labour list, improved monitoring, increased awareness and the creation of special funds to prevent child labour and to support children withdrawn from hazardous child labour.

The Time Bound Programme was formally evaluated in May 2007 by ILO/IPEC and the accomplishments recorded [17]. The evaluation reported that poverty remained the major factor responsible for child labour. A recommendation was made for further improving the incomes of families likely to send their children with supported income-generating activities.

Education, training, and awareness-raising results

The various education measures resulted in some 50,000 children, half of whom were girls, being removed from the worst forms of child labour, and supported to attend education and training. In over 125 primary schools, children at risk of leaving school were supported to stay in school and some 10,000 parents provided with income-generating activities. Local committees were established and assisted in the identification of community resources to support children to stay in schools [17]. The government reviewed all vocational training programmes to match them to current labour demands [18]. However, implementation of training programmes remains a problem.

A cash transfer fund was created targeting families taking care of AIDS-related orphans. According to information coming from Ministry of Gender, Children and Social Development, cash transfer started with 500 households in 2005 in three districts. By December 2008, it covered 25,000 households taking care of more than 75,000 orphans and vulnerable children in 37 districts. It is estimated that by 2012 it will cover 150,000 households and taking care of 450,000 OVCs, where 45% are AIDS-related orphans [17].

Research and monitoring results

The Integrated Household Budget Survey of 2005–2006 provides accurate child labour data to guide and monitor the impact of interventions [5]. Using these data, the government has sought to incorporate child labour into its poverty reduction and jobs creation programmes. A teaching module on child labour has also been introduced for postgraduate students at the University of Nairobi [6].

Rehabilitation of children involved in child labour

Of the children who were removed from the worst forms of child labour under the Time Bound Programme, some were returned to school while others were sent for skills training [16, 18]. Unfortunately many of the courses and equipment used for training children who had been withdrawn from child labour were outdated and did not meet the demands of the market. The duration for training was too long even though most of the children withdrawn came from economically challenged families. Rehabilitating withdrawn children was also a challenge due to lack of safety places where they could temporarily stay while attending training.

Sustainability

While some action programmes recorded successful, sustaining them was a challenge and many programmes ceased to exist beyond the ILO/IPEC Programme. Income-generating activities both in schools and within families did meet with some success as it addressed both poverty at family level and sustainability. Most of the activities were, however, of horticultural nature, and therefore also depended upon the weather: when the rains failed, the crops failed.

Linking the many different actions to existing poverty reduction programmes in the country was challenging and created problems with coordination. Many new action programmes lasted just 1 to 2 years. Established poverty reduction programmes tended to target families which were already organized and committed to change. This meant that the majority of families with children engaged in or at risk of engaging in hazardous child labour were at the mercy of their own limited resources or those of the Time Bound Programme. Support for families to start income-generating activities was most challenged due to the extent of poverty levels and levels of education. Many children withdrawn could not be sustained in school. Lack of food emerged as a major challenge both at home and at school: many children leave home without eating and schools do not provide food.

Conclusions

Current available information indicates that child labour remains widespread in Kenya and is the result mainly of poverty. Many children work in agriculture, domestic service, commercial sexual exploitation, and in the streets. Weak institutions perpetuate the existence of child labour. Although awareness levels of the need to send children to school instead of to work were very low, this has improved considerably among policy makers, service providers, the media, as well as children themselves. A study conducted in 2007 indicated that 60% of the respondents were aware of laws and regulations related to children [17]. All this has resulted from intensive media coverage on child labour in the country.

Major initiatives have now been established to combat child labour in the country starting in 1992 through ILO/IPEC Programme. The government has gone further and developed policies and enacted legislation to fight child labour. The implementation of policies and enforcement of laws remains a challenge. The government, through the Ministry of Labour and Human Resource Development, developed a 15-year National Plan of Action. Implementation of this plan is ongoing. In addition, the government has initiated a number of education policies, and free primary education is being implemented.

Similarly, a number of economic measures have been undertaken through poverty reduction programmes, such as the Economic Recovery Strategy for wealth and employment creation, as well as the 2030 Vision for Kenya. The government has also created bursary and constituency development funds specifically to support children from poor families [18].

Unfortunately, much of the programme has relied upon the leadership of ILO/IPEC; this in turn has created a major challenge of ownership and sustainability. Poverty at the family level is so high that many families in rural and urban areas still find it difficult to educate their children. The availability of food at home and in school has been identified as a determinant factor in child labour currently. The programme may have had some success, but the challenges remain considerable.

References

1 Bwibo NO, Onyango P (1987). The final report of the child labour and health research, ANPPCAN, Nairobi, Kenya.

2 CBS (2001). The 1998/99 Child Labour Report, Nairobi, Kenya.

3 UN Kenya Country Team (2008). UN Development Assistance Framework (UNDAF) 2009–2013.

4 UNICEF (2007). Review of progress towards the world fit for children +5, March 2007.

5 Republic of Kenya (2008). Kenya Integrated Household Budget Survey: Child Labour Analytical Report; Kenya National Bureau of Statistics, Nairobi, Kenya.
6 ILO/IPEC (2009). Project of Support to the National Plan of Action on Elimination of Child Labour in Kenya, January to April 2009, Nairobi, Kenya
7 *Pinnacle Development Consultants (2002):* Baseline Survey on Child Labour in Commercial Agriculture in Kenya, ILO/IPEC, Nairobi.
8 Omosa M, Ontita E, OmbatiH (2004). A rapid assessment of the situation of child domestic workers in Kenya. Nairobi: ILO/IPEC.
9 Onyango P (2004). Rapid assessment on commercial sexual exploitation of children, Nairobi: ILO/IPEC.
10 Republic of Kenya (2003). Report of the Task Force on Implementation of Free Primary Education; Ministry of Education, Science and Technology, Nairobi, Kenya.
11 ILO/IPEC (2003). Taking Stock of Achievements and Lessons Learned. A Report of a Review of IPEC Action Against Child Labour in Kenya 1992–2002, ILO/IPEC Office, Nairobi, Kenya.
12 Republic of Kenya (2002). The Children's Act, 2001, Nairobi, Kenya.
13 Republic of Kenya (2007). The Employment Act 2007, Nairobi, Kenya.
14 MOLHRD (2004). The National Plan of Action on the Elimination of Child Labour in Kenya, 2004–2015, Ministry of Labour and Human Resource Development, Nairobi, Kenya.
15 Republic of Kenya (2004). National Plan of Action on the Elimination of the Worst Forms of child Labour in Kenya, Nairobi, Kenya.
16 Republic of Kenya (2005). Kenya Education Sector Support Programme 2005–2010, Ministry of Education, Science and Technology, Nairobi, Kenya.
17 ILO (2007). Decent Work Kenya: ILO's Country Programme for the Republic of Kenya, 2007–2010.
18 Republic of Kenya (2005). A Policy Framework for Education, Training and Research, Ministry of Education, Science and Technology, Nairobi, Kenya.
19 MOLHRD (2006). National Policy on Child Labour: Towards a Child Labour Free Society, Nairobi, Kenya.
20 Zivetz L, Rutere SK (2009). Final Evaluation Report of the ILO/IPEC Project of support to Time Bound Programme in Kenya.

Chapter 12

Country-wide case studies: The Philippines – A focus on partnerships

Amaryllis T. Torres

Introduction

Child labour in the Philippines includes by statute the employment of children below 15 years of age except in cases of light work under the supervision of parents or guardians, and the employment of young people aged less than 18 years in hazardous occupations [1]. Children work in a range of situations and conditions, paid and unpaid, with remuneration sometimes made directly to adults, or even delivered in non-material ways, such as food, education, shelter, or clothing [2].

This chapter is the third of three county-wide case studies examining the impact of national child labour policies in the context of the public health model of child labour discussed throughout this volume. This Philippine case study focuses on the many partnerships that can be developed to tackle child labour and includes discussion on the impact of the International Labour Organization/International Program on the Elimination of Child Labour (ILO/IPEC) sponsored Philippine Time Bound Project. In terms of the model of child labour, the emphasis in the Philippines has been on legislation, measures to address social values, and most especially on education initiatives.

Child labour in the Philippines

A 2001 survey reported that of 10.4 million Filipino households, a quarter had children working in household-operated enterprises either at home or in other households [3]. Two-thirds of these enterprises were in agriculture and one-third in services. Most working children were aged over 10 years, with a median age of 14–15 years. A total of 4.18 million children worked under these circumstances with boys outnumbering girls by two to one in both urban and rural areas. The 2001 survey figure constituted 16.2% of the total population of children and was higher than it was in 1995 (16% or 3.6 million children).

Of those working, around two-thirds worked in their own household farms or businesses, 21% worked in private establishments, 9.3% worked in private households, and 4.4% were self-employed. Twice as many more boys than girls worked in agriculture, hunting, forestry, and fishing, while more than half of service occupations were held by girls. A quarter of the children worked the whole year; the rest worked either only during the summer vacation, or had short-term casual jobs. A majority (66%) combined schooling with working. On average, children worked for 1 to 4 hours daily, for 3½ days in a week. However, girls were more likely to work longer hours and for more days a week.

Households with working children fared less well on economic indicators (income and expenditure, housing characteristics, and household amenities) than households without working children. The most common reasons given by the children for working were to help in the family business and to augment family income. Less than 10% of both boys and girls said they worked in order to gain experience, acquire training, or learn the value of work.

While the intensity of most child work may be moderate, the risks are high. More than half of the working children had been exposed to hazardous environments including physical, biological, and chemical hazards. It was based on these data that the Philippines formulated a Strategic Framework and Programme to address the worst forms of child labour.

National policy measures to address child labour in the Philippines

Policy and legislative change

The Philippine National Programme against Child Labour (NPACL, 2000–2004) set out to build on more than 20 years of multi-agency efforts to address child labour [4]. The Programme sought to implement international agreements, national laws, policies, and directives to eliminate child labour, to increase knowledge and awareness about child labour, to mobilize social partners from government, civil society, the communities, and families, and thereby to eliminate the worst forms of child labour [5]. Six priority sectors were identified: agriculture, deep-sea fishing, mining and quarrying, pyrotechnics, child prostitution, and domestic work [6].

There were five component parts to the National Programme [4]: Activities under the Philippine ILO/IPEC Time Bound Programme and the ABK

Education Initiative Programme;[1] government-led anti-child labour programmes and projects; UNICEF activities funded through the 5th and 6th Country Programmes for Children; projects undertaken by WINROCK International and projects initiated by non-governmental stakeholders outside of the Time Bound Programme.

The National Programme against Child Labour was implemented through a multi-sectoral, multi-level coordinating body, with the Department of Labour and Employment as the lead agency. Programme implementation committees were newly created or strengthened at city, municipal, and provincial levels where child labour rescue teams were also established.

A number of partnerships with stakeholders from government, civil society, and the private sector were established. The police department and the bureau of immigration were also mobilized, especially for rescue operations and for the enforcement of legal sanctions [4].

New legislation to tackle child labour directly and indirectly was introduced. A national law against Child Labour (Republic Act 9231 or RA 9231), Special Protection of Children against Child Abuse, Exploitation and Discrimination Act) incorporating the provisions of ILO Convention 182 was enacted in 2003. Other national legislation also indirectly addressed child labour: the 2002 Act to Eliminate Trafficking in Persons, Especially Women and Children (RA 9208), and the Anti-Violence against Women and their Children Act of 2004 (RA 9262). Local by-laws addressing child labour were also passed and child labour issues were mainstreamed into the Philippine Medium Term Development Plan.

The Philippine ILO-IPEC Time Bound Programme

The Time Bound Programme was adopted with the aim of eliminating the worst forms of child labour within a defined period of time through combined sectoral, thematic, and geographic approaches. At a preventive level, the Time Bound Programme sought to influence the development of economic and social policies including macro-economic policies, population programmes, and educational and labour market policies. At an intervention level, the Time Bound Programme engaged the State at various levels to assume responsibility for eliminating the worst forms of child labour and mobilized stakeholders on child labour issues. It was on this basis that the National Child Labour

[1] The letters ABK were taken from the three letters of the old Filipino alphabet Alibata to form the acronym for Pag-Aaral ng Bata para sa Kinabukasan (Education for the Children's Future)

Committee set a target of a 75% reduction of the worst forms of child labour by 2015. Under the auspices of the Philippine Time Bound Programme, local government units, communities, and civil society groups committed to the elimination of child labour through a series of memoranda of understanding and resolutions.

In order to identify child workers engaged in hazardous work, a baseline survey was undertaken in eight provinces and in the National Capital Region – all previously identified as having a high incidence of child labour. A total of 103,000 children were located in the nine study sites. Of these, at least 24,000 children worked in any one of the six sectors identified as the worst forms of child labour. To meet the project's target of identifying 45,000 child workers, an additional 21,000 children were selected from the 3000 siblings of working children, and 22,000 other children at-risk in the same geographic areas [7]. Children were selected from this group for educational assistance.

Education projects consisted of new education policies and programmes that included child labour, the mobilization of support from government and non-government institutions, training in child labour issues for teachers, educational assistance to workers' groups, improved access for child workers to alternative and innovative education methods, vocational training, and direct financial assistance for school fees, travel, uniforms, and other educational requirements.

Social values

An employers' confederation promoted many direct services for children: a 'return-to-school' programme, health care services, vocational skills training, and alternative education. It also gave awards to companies recognized as child-labour free and child-friendly. A coalition was formed between employers, trained women, and young people to monitor companies' compliance to standards, to act as an advocate for the inclusion of anti-child labour provisions in collective bargaining agreements, and to monitor child trafficking activities. Workers' organizations and employers both undertook massive advocacy activities within their ranks to campaign against child labour.

Parents' Associations were organized by some social partners (notably the NGOs) to implement livelihood projects. Participatory approaches were applied to empower families of child labourers to analyse their situation, appreciate and mobilize resources. Community organizers undertook measures to raise the awareness of families about child labour, children's rights, and other human rights. The implementation and management of livelihood projects became the responsibility of these organized groups.

The impact of national policy measures to address child labour in the Philippines

Evidence for the impact of the Programme comes from a participatory rapid appraisal undertaken from March to June 2007.[2]

Policy and legislative change

The legal framework to combat child labour was improved with a new National Law, related Acts to tackle trafficking and violence against children, and local codes of practice. Unfortunately, however, there was generally weak enforcement of the new legislation. Poor implementation and a slow legal process were common problems, and efforts were sometimes thwarted because of legal procedural impediments. For example, it took up to five years from the rescue of some children to the sentencing of the culprits. Political influence benefited establishments employing minors (notably 'commercially and sexually exploited children') and prosecution was difficult: many cases against traffickers and perpetuators were not even filed. In extreme cases, the alleged perpetrator became the plaintiff against the person responsible for his/her apprehension.

Education

Educational support was provided to child workers through the ABK Education Initiative, the Time Bound Programme and WINROCK International.

The ABK Education Initiative provided educational subsidies to 31,000 male and female children, 54% of whom were child labourers and 46% children at risk of becoming child labourers. More than two-thirds of those assisted were involved in the agriculture sector, principally in sugar production. As a result of ABK's support, 54% of identified child workers were withdrawn from work, with an approximately equal numbers of boys and girls [8].

Children working in quarrying, children who were commercially and sexually exploited, and child domestic workers appeared to be least able to access ABK services. This may have been because ABK partners were not present in the villages where most quarrying took place, and both domestic workers and commercial and sexually exploited children are highly mobile. Even in the Capital where commercially and sexually exploited children were surveyed, it

[2] The National Programme against Child Labour was complex and multi-dimensional. It was implemented by many agencies at various levels of society in pursuit of different strategic goals. Only key aspects of the programme evaluation are described here in keeping with the purposes of this section of the book.

is likely that employers and pimps hid children or forced them to move and work elsewhere to avoid being detected.

ABK developed several support mechanisms. These included a field manual for monitoring child labour, community watch groups to monitor school attendance, a national children's association with opportunities for child workers to participate in innovative educational programmes, and assistance to parents of child beneficiaries [9].

Education interventions also constituted a major aspect of the ILO/IPEC Philippine Time Bound Programme. As a result of the ILO/IPEC Time Bound Programme, 40,549 child workers were assisted (Table 12.1). The parents of 1782 children at risk of being employed in deep-sea fishing and 2634 children in sugar plantations were provided with financial support on the condition of school enrolment. Children rescued from trafficking were provided with educational support, vocational skills training, training in information technology, sewing, crocheting, food processing, and cooking. In the Autonomous Region of Muslim Mindanao, 120 former child soldiers and other children at risk were enrolled in formal school, while 277 were given vocational or non-formal courses. Graduates were then assisted to find work overseas, while 115 graduates in sugar production technology were hired by sugar mills [10].

WINROCK International undertook a series of educational initiatives through its Community-based Innovations to Reduce Child Labor through Education project (CIRCLE). WINROCK had five partner organizations in its CIRCLE project from 2004 to 2006, and targeted 902 child workers or children at risk of the worst forms of child labour. At the end of the project, services had been provided to 979 children [11].

The project's innovative methods included child-to-child programmes, parent–teacher focus groups; and peer pressure teams who kept records on school attendance. WINROCK's projects also had an impact on local planning processes. For example, the evaluation information it collated was utilized by the Barangay Committees for the Protection of Children to develop their own programmes. In some instances this led to local legislation for child protection (e.g. curfew hours, sanctions against employers of child workers) and to improved health and safety provisions.

As a result of ABK, WINROCK, and ILO/IPEC's various schemes of assistance, there was an increase in children's enrolment and attendance, better school performance, improved retention and completion rates and improved employment opportunities [4, 9, 12]. It was also noted that being in school helped to prevent child workers from sliding back into other worst forms of child labour, such as prostitution [13]. Field interviews and observations, however, demonstrated that these educational initiatives did not eliminate child labour. Instead children spent less time at work and more time at school.

Table 12.1 Number and percentage of children withdrawn or prevented from WFCL: ILO-IPEC PTBP, by sectors, total project duration (as of August 2006)

Sector of WFCL	Status	education services or training		other non-education services		total number of children	
		Boys	**Girls**	**Boys**	**Girls**	***F***	**%*Total***
Sugar plantations	Withdrawn	5976	4445	1514	724	12659	31.2
	Prevented	2717	2305	838	1074	6934	17.0
Child domestic labour	Withdrawn	607	1484	509	2508	4658	11.5
	Prevented	998	1425	272	529	3224	8.0
Deep sea fishing	Withdrawn	818	198	117	60	1193	2.9
	Prevented	1512	1147	144	204	3007	7.4
Pyrotechnics	Withdrawn	700	631	368	328	2027	5.0
	Prevented	316	248	820	706	2090	5.2
Commercial sexual exploitation children	Withdrawn	361	777	302	410	1850	4.6
	Prevented	177	396	186	186	945	2.3
Mining & quarrying	Withdrawn	891	537	38	21	1487	3.7
	Prevented	178	201	49	47	475	1.2
Total number of child-beneficiaries, by sex		15,251	13,794	5,157	6,347	40,549	100%
Total number of child-beneficiaries, by type of programme		29,045		11,504		TOTAL = 40,549	

There were also difficulties with inadequate resources in the public school system, such as classroom and teacher shortages. Moreover, the financial resources allotted to educational assistance were meagre (ranging from £1.4 to £7 per pupil per year) compared to actual expenses for schooling, and were largely confined to school supplies and uniforms. Very few college scholarships were available, so that at 16 years of age, most high school graduates could not find regular employment. Thus, some of the children went back to work while others remained idle [4].

Rescue programmes

Established in 1993 after the successful rescue of child workers from a sardines canning factory, the *Sagip Bata Manggagawa* (Child Labour Rescue) Quick Action Teams (SBM-QAT) are community-based teams which detect, monitor, and report on the most intolerable forms of child labour [14]. In 1994 a memorandum of understanding was forged between *Sagip-Bata Manggagawa*, government agencies, two trade unions, one employers' group and two non-government organizations [15]. The SBM-QAT remains in place to this day.

In a 2006 report to a Committee of Experts on the Application of Conventions and Recommendations, it was recorded that between 1998 and 2005, 1761 children (including 847 females) were rescued from the worst forms of child labour. Consequently, four criminal cases were filed against employers found in breach of national legislation [15].

Despite some success, however, a chronic lack of funds for operations limits search and rescue operations, subsequent legal proceedings, and the provision of support for rescued children. Furthermore, the SBM-QAT's mandate ends with rescue and many court cases against offenders have been dismissed due to lack of evidence, corruption, or because parents and their children withdrew from the cases.

Micro-economic and other measures

School participation and withdrawal from work were often made as conditions to accessing economic programmes. At the time of the programme assessment, around 7042 families of child workers had been given livelihood assistance through micro-credit, basic literacy, and vocational and income-generating skills. A total of 4471 families reported an increase in their income as a result of this assistance [15]. Most of these assisted families worked in agriculture communities – principally sugar plantations, deep-sea fishing, pyrotechnics, mining, and quarrying. Families of commercially and sexually exploited children and child domestic workers were more difficult to find and engage.

Livelihood skills training did not always guarantee increased income because of limited employment opportunities. Seasonal demand for certain skills left many adults with periods of no income, which may have resulted in children looking for work. Poor links between skills development, credit schemes, and markets threatened the sustainability of small enterprises.

Some small gains were made through economic assistance programmes with some children completely released from the necessity to work. More often than not, however, there remained the possibility of children's participation in labour, especially when adult work was insufficiently secure to provide for the household.

In addition to education and financial assistance, a variety of interventions such as health and nutrition programmes, legal assistance, help desks and hotlines, repatriation assistance, temporary shelter, and psycho-social counselling were also provided. Towards the end of the National Programme, social protection programmes, community-based insurance schemes, and community enterprise developments were also established. Field accounts report that success and sustainability were more likely where there was cooperation and coordination of different interventions.

Conclusions

A total of 73,619 children were withdrawn from child labour or prevented from taking it up as a result of the National Programme [8, 11, 15]. This number exceeded the programme target which was set at 44,500 child workers. More than half of the assisted children were girls.

Despite this success, a number of important gaps were identified in the National Programme. The children who obtained assistance were concentrated in the project areas of the National Programme's partners. Although the target was exceeded, the number of children who were assisted still constitutes a small proportion of working children, even with regard to just those in the worst forms.

Educational programmes did not eliminate child labour but rather resulted in the temporary removal of children from hazardous work. At best, educational support enabled children to disengage from hazardous work, spend more hours in school and fewer hours at work, complete basic education, acquire skills, and improve their chances of getting better employment as adults. A system for monitoring school attendance, retention, and completion would assist in assessing the effects of education programmes.

Many of the initiatives were solely dependent on project funds and faced problems of continuity and sustainability. Improved implementation and enforcement of policy and legislation were also required, as well as increased government commitment to forge wider partnerships. Programmes and services for children need to address not just child labour, but also health, education, shelter safety, and personal security.

There were successes, and if properly resourced, the Philippines National Programme as a model to effectively tackle child labour does have some merit. Key to any approach, and what is reflected in the child labour model discussed throughout this volume, is that tackling child labour effectively requires multiple interventions. Thus, the collaborative effort of different stakeholders, organizations, and communities constitutes a key element in reducing the harm that children experience from working.

References

1 ILS–DOLE (1994). Comprehensive study on child labor in the Philippines Institute of Labor Studies, Department of Labor and Employment, Manila, Philippines.

2 Tiglao-Torres, A (2002). Rapid appraisal of child labor in the tobacco industry: Case studies in two Ilocos provinces. PARTNERS INTL Inc. Child Protection in the Philippines: Philippine Resource Network; Available at http://www.childprotection.org.ph/monthlyfeatures/archives/aug2k5a.html; Also in Eliminating Child Labor: ECLT Foundation. Available at www.eclt.org/filestore/PARTNERS_Appraisal_CL_Tobacco_Philippines.pdf.

3 NSO & ILO-IPEC (2003). *2001 Survey of Children 5–17 years old*. ILO, Manila, Philippines.

4 Torres, Amaryllis (2007). Nurturing children for a better future: gains and prospects from the national program against child labor: final report on the performance assessment of the NPACL. Final Report. National Program against Child Labor: Manila, Philippines.

5 Bureau of Women and Young Workers, Department of Labor and Employment (BWYW-DOLE). NPACL framework. *National program against child labor (2000–2004)*. Available at http://www.bwyw.dole.gov.ph (accessed January 2007).

6 BWYW (2001). *National program against child labor: Strategic pans 2001–2004*. BWYW: Manila, Philippines.

7 Resurreccion, Angelita (2006). Time-bound programme baseline survey: integrative report. ILO-IPEC, Makati, Philippines.

8 ABK Monitoring and Evaluation MIS (2007). *Gender Cohort Analysis*. ABK Education Initiative: QC, Philippines.

9 ABK Education Initiative (2003). Technical reference for effective information management in project implementation of child labor education initiative. *ABK field manual*. QC, Philippines.

10 ILO-IPEC (2006). Time bound programme project update. Makati, Philippines.

11 WINROCK International and CIRCLE SEA Available at http://circle.winrock.org/circle_asia.cfm (accessed May 2007).

12 Frankel, N (2005). *Evaluation of ABK Initiative in the Philippines*. Development Associates: Virginia, USA.

13 Pacis, Roland (2002). An in-depth study for a time-bound program targeting child domestic workers in the Philippines. ILO-IPEC, Manila.

14 KDF. Municipality of Kananga, Leyte. Kamalayan Development Foundation. Available at http://kananga.blogs.friendster.com/my_blog/2007/05/kamalayan_devel.html (accessed 29 May 2007).

15 ILO-IPEC (March 2004; September 2004; March 2005; September 2005; March 2006; September 2006; March 2007). Technical progress reports, ILO-IPEC, Makati, Philippines.

Chapter 12A

Illustrative case study A: A child labour monitoring programme: RugMark

Nina Smith

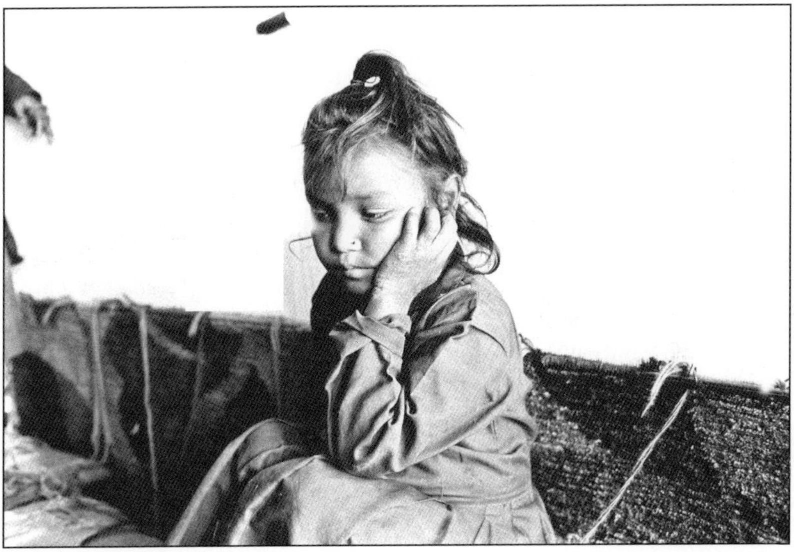

Carpet weaver, Nepal

Introduction

Handmade rugs are among South Asia's top export products. In the hands of skilled adult artisans, handmade rugs are true cultural expressions and works of art; far too often, however, they are made by exploited children. Children aged 4–14 years are kidnapped or sold into debt bondage and forced labour on carpet looms. They are subject to malnutrition, impaired vision, and deformities from sitting long hours in cramped loom sheds.

Tragically, their labour helps ensure that their own children will suffer the same fate. A 2008 study conducted by Evidence, an Indian human rights organization, reveals that the parents of 85% of children surveyed were also labourers during their childhood [1]. Laws against child labour in South Asian producer countries exist, but are not enforced.

In 1994, United Nations Children's Fund (UNICEF), the International Labour Organization (ILO), the Indo-German Export Promotion Program and the South Asian Coalition on Child Servitude, which represents 250 NGOs, joined together to take a new approach. RugMark was founded as one of the world's first independent labour monitoring programs, designed to drive both supply and demand for child-labour-free rugs while providing comprehensive educational and rehabilitation opportunities for rescued and at-risk children.

RugMark is based on a simple premise: If enough people demand certified child-labour-free rugs, manufacturers will only employ skilled, adult artisans and the exploitation of children in the carpet industry will come to an end. RugMark catalyses this industry-wide transformation by certifying and promoting rugs with the GoodWeave (formerly RugMark) label[1] – proof that they were made by a fairly employed adult. To date, more than six million carpets bearing the RugMark label have been sold in Europe and North America.

At the time of RugMark's launch, an estimated one million South Asian children were trapped in illegal and exploitative carpet-making work. Today, largely due to RugMark's efforts, that number stands at an estimated 250,000 [2, 3]. This chapter explores how RugMark has succeeded in a broad range of social and economic initiatives designed to ultimately eradicate child labour in the handmade rug industry, while providing a powerful model for other child labour efforts.

RugMark's Origins

World-wide attention was drawn to the use of child labour in handmade rugs in the 1980s and early 1990s. Studies by the ILO [4], the US Department of Labour; [5] and human rights groups[6,7,8] [6–8] revealed that the industry was illegally employing and exploiting large numbers of children. Many were found to be victims of debt bondage or forced labour, practices specifically banned by the United Nations and the ILO and condemned as contemporary forms of slavery.

By the late 1980s, Kailash Satyarthi, chairman of the South Asian Coalition on Child Servitude and a leader in the fight against child labour, wanted to create a market incentive for manufacturers to stop exploiting children on an industry-wide basis. In September 1994, he founded the RugMark Foundation. The first carpets bearing the certification label were exported from India at the beginning

1 In 2009 RugMark International re-branded its certification label to GoodWeave to better reflect the meaning behind the label and to position the organization to move into new manufacturing sectors where child labour exists and can be eliminated through market change.

of 1995, mainly to Germany. Since then, additional operations have taken hold in Nepal (a producer nation) and the US and UK (importing nations).

The RugMark approach

RugMark International (RMI) is the governing body of each national RugMark initiative. A members' council made up of representatives from each of the five RugMark chapters sets policies and ensures national-level accountability. RMI is a member of the International Social and Environmental Accreditation and Labelling Alliance (ISEAL), an independent alliance that works to ensure the effectiveness and credibility of social/environmental standard-setting organizations. RugMark is working towards meeting ISEAL's code of best practice, which represents the alliance's highest governing standards for transparency, accountability, and stakeholder engagement.

RugMark International's work involves: monitoring and certification; child rescue, rehabilitation and education; and building a marketplace where the certification is demanded and available.

Monitoring and Certification

Companies that join RugMark and meet its strict no-child-labour standards (no children under the age of 14 employed) are issued certification labels for their carpets. To protect against counterfeit labeling, each label is numbered so its origin can be traced back to the loom on which the rug was produced.

Inspectors trained and supervised by RugMark pay unannounced visit to licensed premises in South Asia. To receive the RugMark certification, manufacturers sign a legally binding contract to:

- produce carpets without illegal child labour;
- register all looms with the RugMark Foundation;
- allow access to looms for unannounced inspections; and
- pay associated license fees.

RugMark believes that ultimately industry should pay for its own regulation and was set up as a self-financing model. US importers that use the RugMark label on their rugs pay RugMark USA a license fee of 1.75% of the export value of shipments. 57% of these fees underwrites social programmes in South Asia, and the balance is invested in Rugmark USA's awareness campaign. Industry fees currently represent 22% of RugMark USA's budget, and are expected to contribute to 50% of the budget by as soon as 2012.

Child rescue and education

Once the licensing process is initiated, RugMark inspects the licensed company's supply chain and rescues every child labourer discovered – more than 3600 to date.

Once children are rescued, RugMark attempts to reunite them with their families. Children are then invited to attend school and with their families decide whether to enroll in a RugMark-affiliated school or to live at home and attend a public or private school with financial support.

Initially, RugMark founded and ran each of its schools independently. This process proved unsustainably demanding over time, however, and RugMark has since shifted to a partnership model: local NGOs and government and private schools provide the educational services, and RugMark plays the role of placing rescued children in a suitable setting and paying for the cost of their education.

Most children rescued from the looms never had an education or dropped out of school at an early age. RugMark programmes begin with intensive literacy and basic math training, preparing them for a formal education. Formal education programmes include language training, social studies, math, and science. Children also enjoy physical fitness and extracurricular pursuits in music and art.

RugMark schools encourage high academic standards, and every effort is made to help children continue their education through high school. Children over age 14 who excel are often transferred to private schools preparing them for higher education. Others are encouraged to join vocational training programmes supported by RugMark, and are assisted in job placement once they reach legal working age.

The RugMark approach also stresses prevention by investing in proactive programmes such as workers' rights workshops, and adult literacy classes. Additionally, RugMark funds initiatives that contribute to healthy, financially independent communities, such as daycare and education for children of adult carpet workers; advocacy and awareness programmes that provide parents with support and information; and mobile medical services for carpet workers and their children.

Building an ethical marketplace

Through social marketing, awareness campaigns, and business development, RugMark is building a marketplace in which child-labour-free rugs are demanded and available. One of the markers of the success of the programme is the number of companies and consumers that select RugMark.

More than 75 rug design and import companies in the US and Canada and 42 companies in Europe participate in RugMark. They include small start-ups and larger, more established companies, with rug designs from traditional to contemporary. The rugs are sold through more than 1500 retail outlets and internet sites in North America.

RugMark works to drive demand for child-labour-free rugs by working cooperatively with retailers and building awareness among socially conscious consumers and the interior design community. Launched in 2005, our 'Most Beautiful Rug' marketing campaign – which emphasized that only a rug made without child labour can be considered beautiful – features increased joint marketing with partner companies in both the import and retail sectors. Advertising and editorial placements, trade and consumer events, and point-of-sale brochures and education are key components, along with GoodWeave.org. The campaign has grown sales of certified rugs by nearly 100% with imports increasing from $7.3 to $13.2 million, or 3.25% market share, in 3 years.

The goal of awareness raising is to gain 7% of the market by 2010 and 15% market share by as soon as 2012. RugMark hypothesizes that 15% market share in the US will trigger the tipping point that ends child labour in South Asia's handmade rug industry. RugMark anticipates accomplishing its tipping point in three phases. The first phase, 'early adoption', has already been completed; Odegard Company became RugMark USA's first licensee and with its CEO led a group of companies who signed with RugMark out of primarily social and ethical concerns.

Now almost every company motivated by these factors alone has joined RugMark. The campaign is currently in Phase Two: retail industry leaders are joining RugMark for economic advantages in addition to moral ones. Plans are underway for a 2010 Macy's partnership, and at least one other industry leader is slated to begin selling GoodWeave-certified rugs this year. In Phase Three, termed 'late adoption', companies that may not ever pursue social issues in their operations will still sign, because of the strong business case that certification presents.

Measuring impact

Several indicators suggest that RugMark is succeeding in its efforts to shift the handmade rug industry toward a child-labour-free standard:

- RugMark licensees are selling more rugs. Despite flat or falling sales in the overall industry, sales by RugMark's top seven licensees increased by 15% from 2006 to 2007. In 2008, industry sales fell 19% and RugMark certified rug sales increased 15%.
- Market growth coincided with the launch of the 'Most Beautiful Rug' campaign. The campaign was introduced with a baseline market share of 1%; that market share grew to 3.25% in 2008.
- In the three years since launching 'The Most Beautiful Rug', the campaign has delivered an average growth of 21% per year.

The impact on communities in producer countries is also promising:

- A decrease in child labour has coincided with RugMark's operations. Data from UNICEF [2] and U.S. Department of State [3] reports show that in RugMark's first decade of operation, child labour on South Asian looms dropped from 1 million to 300,000 as market share grew to 1.5%.
- Field staff in Nepal report that local attitudes about the value of educating children are changing. Parents of children who have benefited from RugMark early childhood education and school-sponsorship programmes are now finding resources to send other siblings and children to school.
- The number of children rescued, rehabilitated, and schooled with RugMark support is growing, though slowly. Since 1995 RugMark inspectors have directly rescued more than 3600 children. In Nepal, 95% of rescued children have opted to receive rehabilitation/schooling.

Conclusion

The success of the RugMark model has far-reaching implications for child labour. Combining education, rehabilitation, and prevention with effective, market-driven strategies is a highly replicable model that can be applied to many other settings and countries.

The model is not universally applicable. There are myriad factors, including civil war, changes in production techniques and locations, and government investments in enforcement and education, that can seriously impact the success of inspection, monitoring, and certification. Nonetheless, it is RugMark's conviction that as long as socially conscious consumers can be made aware of the impact of their purchases, market-driven reform can succeed where laws and societal infrastructure fail.

Reference

1 5 US Department of Labor, Bureau of International Labor Affairs (15 July 1994). By the sweat and toil of children: The use of child labor in American imports. Available at http://www.dol.gov/ILAB/media/reports/iclp/sweat/sweat.pdf (accessed 30 June 2009).

Chapter 12B

Illustrative case study B: Applying agricultural work guidelines from one country in another

Barbara C. Lee

Introduction

Worldwide, agriculture is the industry most likely to involve children as workers [1]. The nature of production agriculture may require work at any time of day, every day of the year, and often in adverse conditions. Besides the unpredictable nature of hot, cold, and stormy weather, complications of outdoor work may include airborne and dermal exposures to chemicals, dusts, bites, and stings from arthropods and reptiles, as well as mammal bites and kicks. Further, water sources such as irrigation ditches and manure pits harbour dangers associated with drowning or ingestion of contaminated fluids [2].

In contrast to typical work settings, there can be vague distinctions between formal labour in agriculture and non-work activities. Children of very young ages may be contributing to productive planting, harvesting, or animal care tasks while working alone or merely accompanying parents/adults in the work setting. In those countries which have applicable child labour regulations, there is limited public knowledge of their existence and minimal oversight or enforcement by regulators [3].

In 1999, the North American Guidelines for Children's Agricultural Tasks (NAGCAT) were released as a new resource to help adults match a child's physical, mental, and psychosocial abilities with the requirements of agricultural jobs [4]. The NAGCAT were developed by a multidisciplinary team from the United States, Canada, and Mexico, using a systematic job hazard analysis process.

The unique feature of NAGCAT is their establishment based upon child growth and development principles in contrast to chronological age. These principles are relatively universal. NAGCAT uses a non-judgmental approach in guiding decisions about work duties, acknowledging parents' perceived value, or need of children's participation in agricultural work. Globally, the reasons for children's work in agriculture are complex and varied. Using child growth and development principles as a basis for work offers the opportunity to identify situations where involvement in appropriate, safe work can be rewarding to children and adults.

Illustrated NAGCAT posters are intended for use by parents of children aged 7 to 16 years, providing valuable opportunities to work in agriculture under the direction of parents or guardians. They are not intended for use when children are hired to work apart from their parents or guardians, and they do not reference any laws or regulations.

Although many resources exist for promoting childhood farm safety, only NAGCAT has undergone intense testing and evaluation which has led to its widespread acceptance. A five-year assessment of NAGCAT's strengths and weaknesses was conducted and future priorities were suggested [5]. The National Institute for Occupational Safety and Health (NIOSH) reported that, in addition to funding the original development of NAGCAT, they funded six independent NAGCAT-related studies from 2000 through 2008 [6].

The most notable study regarding the efficacy of these guidelines was conducted by Gadomski and colleagues [7]. In central New York State, 845 farm households with children were randomized to a NAGCAT intervention group or to a control group. Outreach educators visited intervention sites to provide and promote use of the guidelines. Data on childhood injuries, tasks, and hours worked were obtained quarterly for 21 months. Injury events were compared between treatment and control groups and then coded to assess whether adherence to the NAGCAT guidelines could have prevented the injury. Results showed that nearly half of all childhood farm injuries could have been prevented had guidelines been followed and, indeed, for the intervention families using the guidelines, there was a 52% reduction in injuries compared to the control group.

Key elements of guidelines for children's agricultural tasks

The paediatric, scientific basis for NAGCAT allows for their adaptation beyond North American agriculture. The very first step in setting guidelines is the identification of jobs or tasks in which children might be involved. Depending on the geographic or commodity-based agriculture, children's work may involve field work, animal handling, small equipment operation, and ambient conditions such as recent spraying of pesticides or increased risk of heat-related illness.

Children physically grow, learn to think, and develop emotionally at their individual pace. Chronological age is rarely an indicator of a child's readiness to be engaged in meaningful work. To develop agricultural work guidelines, the growth and development characteristics of children must be applied to the various tasks associated with a given job.

Let us take the example of a job that requires close contact with cows or pigs. First, it is essential that the child be able to respond quickly to animal behaviour. At about ages 7 to 9 years, most children have a slow reaction time, tire quickly, and easily get bored. By age 10 to 11, a child's attention span may increase to 20 minutes, but they may still lack a sense of awareness of their surroundings. Overall, adolescents' behaviour is unpredictable and, typically, girls mature sooner than boys. All adolescents have a growing sense of responsibility and could be trained to understand animal instinctive behaviours. With training, personal protective equipment, and supervision, adolescents can safely conduct many agricultural work assignments (Table 12B.1)

Sixty-two NAGCAT illustrated posters and background criteria are available online (www.nagcat.org). Each established guideline has anywhere from 6 to 23 steps to complete the job. These are followed by a checklist of adult responsibilities, a listing of hazards, important steps to remember, and then a series of yes/no/STOP questions pertinent to the child's developmental characteristics associated with those variables.

Many NAGCAT guidelines, such as hand harvesting fruits and vegetables, cleaning grain bins, catching and holding a pig, or repairing a fence, have aspects that are common to a multitude of agricultural jobs in various geographic regions and commodity-based agricultural sites. By starting with the job hazard analysis framework of an established NAGCAT task, the core content for a new guideline, addressing a local need, can readily be developed via modification or customization. The process will require: (1) selecting a job (e.g. harvesting rice), (2) listing in sequence the steps for getting the job done, (3) identifying and reviewing current NAGCAT jobs with similar steps, (4) identifying main hazards, injury/disease concerns, recommended procedures (e.g. protective footwear), training required, and ideal level of supervision for each step, (5) referring to NAGCAT for related child development principles, and (6) compiling the core content for that job into a reference document in chart or narrative form.

Once the new core content is deemed accurate and relevant, the next step is to portray and disseminate the information in a culturally, linguistically, and socially acceptable manner. The original NAGCAT includes individually developed illustrations that depict a job being done correctly, as well as illustrations that feature points to remember (e.g. water jug emphasizing need to maintain adequate hydration). Illustrations can be more advantageous than photographs since ideal conditions can be ensured. In contrast, it is difficult to

Table 12B.1 Child growth and development principles applied to work assignments

Growth and development characteristics	Implications for work
Age 7 to 9 years	
Growth and development characteristics	**Implications for work**
Children cannot easily remember job tasks from situation to situation or day to day	Show and tell children each time you want a job done
Children have poor eye–hand coordination; attention span is about 12 minutes; they have boundless energy	Give short, easily completed jobs
Children have a slow reaction time	Avoid jobs that require quick response (e.g. animals that kick)
Children learn by watching other people's behaviors	Set and enforce safety rules then model safe behavior
Ages 10 to 11 years	
Growth and development characteristics	**Implications for work**
Children learn by seeing how it is done	Show and tell children each time how to do the job
Attention span is about 20 minutes	Give jobs of short duration
Children are becoming more independent from families and more influenced by peers	Set and enforce consistent rules and provide close supervision
During a rapid growth spurt, there may be muscle and joint strain leading to decreased coordination	Limit jobs that put excessive strain on joints such as heavy lifting or repetitive tasks
Females typically reach puberty up to two years earlier than males	Be aware of different levels of coordination based on gender when assigning jobs
Ages 12 to 13 years	
Growth and development characteristics	**Implications for work**
As peers become more important, adolescents may try unsafe things to get attention	Set and enforce consistent rules and give praise for safe behaviors
Rebellious, risk taking behavior and perception of immortality puts adolescents at risk	Consistently role model safe practices and provide adequate supervision
Adolescents primarily focus on themselves and behavior is unpredictable	Reassess job assignments frequently
Boys may experience puberty with growth spurts leading to clumsiness	Be alert for decreased coordination and limit jobs that put excessive strain on joints, such as heavy, repetitive lifting
Ages 14 to 15 years	
Growth and development characteristics	**Implications for work**
Certain jobs become easier and quality of work is better as strength and coordination improves	Slowly increase the complexity of jobs

Table 12B.1 (*Cont'd*) Child growth and development principles applied to work assignments

Growth and development characteristics	Implications for work
As adolescents struggle between adulthood and childhood, behavior is unpredictable	Increase supervision with more complex jobs
Boys may still be going through rapid growth spurts	Be alert for decreased coordination and limit jobs that put excessive strain on joints
Rebellious, risk taking behaviors increases risk of injury	Set and enforce consistent rule
Ages 16 to 18 years	
Growth and development characteristics	**Implications for work**
Adolescents have increased ability to think and understand a concept without seeing it	Describe jobs and demonstrate new tasks
Adolescents may believe their size and age predict ability	Provide adequate supervision based on child's abilities and behavior patterns

Modified from Child Development Chart, North American Guidelines for Children's Agricultural Tasks, Professional Resource Manual [Reference 4], pp. 8–10

capture on camera, a job being done appropriately, taking into account all recommended conditions for the worker and the environment. Further, illustrations can range from quite simplistic or elaborate and be matched to the style or preference commonly used by the end-user. In cases where non-visual guidelines are disseminated, audio or videotape lessons or storytelling approaches can be used.

Applications for adolescents hired to work in agriculture

Upon request from United States agricultural employers who hire teenagers, new resources were developed and released in 2008. Safety Guidelines for Hired Adolescent Farm Workers are appropriate for situations where young adults are legally employed to conduct agricultural work [8]. These resources, derived from the original NAGCAT, are available with a supervisor's training manual, addressing seven topics: adolescents at work, outdoor work, basic tractor operations, hand fruits and vegetables, harvesting tree fruit and climbing a ladder, working with large animals, and working with utility vehicles [9]. The illustrated guidelines (in English and Spanish) depict ideal working conditions, teen assessment, training and supervision, and pertinent US federal regulations. These guidelines are valid in situations where US Child Labor in Agriculture Regulations apply [10]. Intervention studies are now underway to motivate labour-intensive agriculture operations to adopt these guidelines for their young hired workforce and for workers with limited English language skills and/or new to agricultural work (Figure 12B.1).

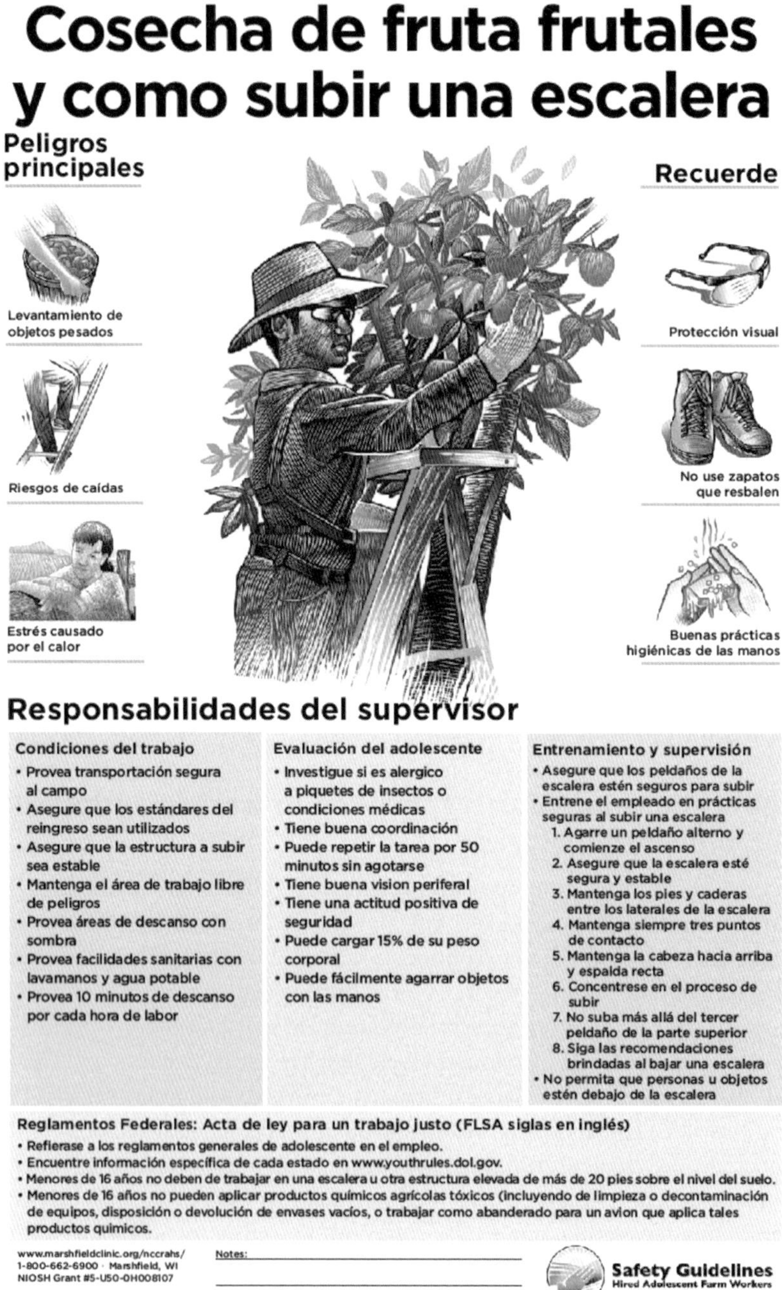

Fig. 12B.1 Illustrated SAGHAF poster, Spanish, Harvesting Tree Fruit

International applications of NAGCAT

The 12-member project team that developed NAGCAT tried to ensure that children working in North American agricultural settings were represented, although conditions in Mexico differed notably from those in the US and Canada. Within a few months of their release, many of the illustrated posters were translated into Spanish and French. These are currently available online (www.nagcat.org) and can be reproduced at no charge. Shortly after their 1999 release, interest was expressed in several countries wanting to adopt the guidelines for specific populations where children were engaged in agricultural work.

Internationally, agricultural practices differ significantly based on many factors, most notably the overall level of development of the country and region. It follows that the types and rates of childhood agriculture-related injuries are closely related to the working conditions of each site. A few examples of how the essential elements of NAGCAT have been adopted in different settings may guide future attempts to apply the basic elements of NAGCAT in developing countries.

In 2008 a team from the University of Wisconsin sought to explore the applicability of Spanish NAGCAT resources in Tepatitlan, Mexico, a region with many dairies and agriculture-related industries (publication forthcoming). The investigative team was fluent in Spanish and had previous experience living in Central America, thus, they adapted well to the region where they were pilot-testing NAGCAT. Their first objective was to determine the most common farm-related injuries among child workers. To do this, they interviewed local physicians, visited clinics, and reviewed emergency room records. Next they visited farms and observed working situations to better understand the tasks performed by children and their inherent risks. They gathered information on hygiene practices, lifting, handling of pesticides, harvesting techniques, types of vehicles used on the site, and safety procedures. Additionally, they documented characteristics of sites where children work, such as number of milk-producing cows, number of acres farmed, and household conditions. Interacting with parents, they solicited information on common injuries or accidents that occur on those farms. Finally, they met with leaders of a local cooperative that sold milk and other products from 26 local farms that had children on site to determine if the cooperative could serve as a facilitator of farm safety education.

The conclusion of this study in Mexico was that children were performing many tasks similar to those on US farms. Medical records were determined to be a weak data source to assess the incidence or prevalence in childhood agricultural injuries. Many injury events and outcomes were the same, such as being kicked or pinned against an object by a cow and suffering a fracture. At the same time, other exposures were unique to the region, including scorpion bites and mushroom poisoning. The leaders of the farm cooperative were very willing to learn, adapt, and promote safety practices among their members. Further, they indicated interest in hosting future visits from individuals who could help them modify NAGCAT for their region. Without such outside support, it is uncertain if this next step will be taken.

Another example that relates to developing nations comes from the metropolitan area of St. Paul, Minnesota (US) where there is a large Hmong population who are recent immigrants from southeast Asia (Laos). Hmong families engage in agricultural practices that are based on traditional practices from their home country. The project team aimed to investigate their agricultural exposures and specific health and safety behaviours in order to guide the development of culturally appropriate health and safety interventions [11]. Hmong children work or play alongside their parents in the field, as well as at the market, where they sell their produce. Gender roles and expectations are shaped by men who hold decision-making positions.

Using a non-experimental approach, Hmong farm families were interviewed to gather information on demographics of Hmong families engaged in agriculture, typical children's tasks, parents' safety knowledge and behaviour, preferred learning methods regarding safety issues, and general reactions to the current NAGCAT guidelines. It was noted that farming practices are generally small-scale operations using mainly hand tools, manual labour, and local direct-marketing sales. For Hmong children, jobs differed by gender and work tasks of all children included use of knives, machetes, digging sticks, and hoes to plant and harvest a variety of fruits, vegetables, and herbs. Gas-powered hand tillers with sharp blades were used to prepare the ground for planting.

Only a few of the available NAGCAT guidelines were specific to the work conducted by Hmong children. Following attempts to translate and modify two printed NAGCAT posters, it was determined that written materials would not be well received. Project leaders working with leaders and mothers within the immigrant community modified their approach to be consistent with the population. In the end, a series of stories were developed to deliver human interest messages that included safety information based on NAGCAT. Stories were initially told by Hmong leaders to children and parents. Over a few years of telling these stories, the messages were refined. Ultimately, they were saved by writing and illustrating each message, which is now available in a children's-style book, *Orphan Boy the Farmer* [12] (Figure 12B.2).

A third example comes from the Philippines where more than two million children work in agriculture. Research revealed that the greatest injury risk factor for children conducting agricultural work was the use of hand

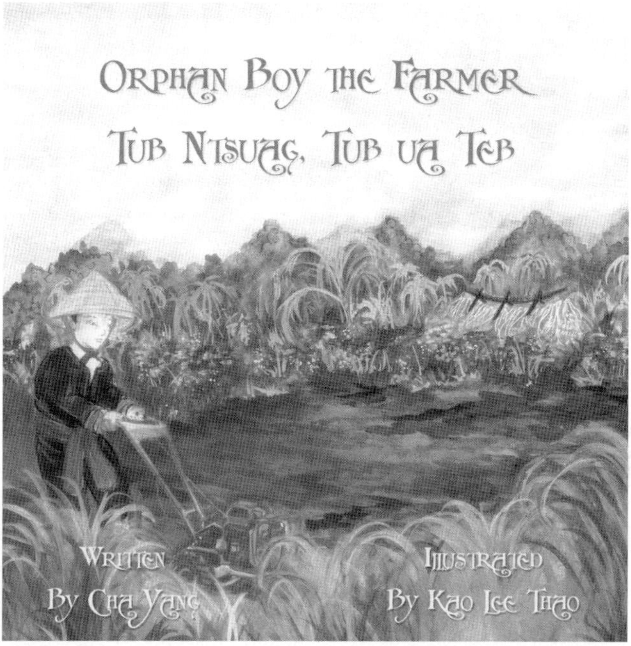

Fig. 12B.2 Book cover of *Orphan Boy the Farmer*, example of Hmong storytelling © Kao Lee and Michele Schermann. Reproduced with kind permission.

tools/equipment [13]. Based on this evidence and the NAGCAT framework, a guideline for harvesting sugarcane was developed (Table 12B.2). The guideline explains how excessive muscle strain from carrying materials can be minimized. It also recommends the use of protective gear, such as sturdy gloves and rubber shoes, to minimize cuts from hand tools and puncture wounds from cane points. Now that this core content is secured, the information can be prepared for dissemination to the target population through visual resources, via verbal instructions, or other locally acceptable methods.

Summary

Where children's participation in agricultural activities is necessary or desired, the role of parents, guardians, and employers as the protectors of child workers cannot be understated. Work guidelines that are developed using sound principles, and which promote best practices, have the potential to change the ways that adults train, supervise, and assign tasks to children making working conditions safer. The North American Guidelines for Children's Agricultural Tasks were developed with the theme of 'helping children do the job safely' and research has confirmed their effectiveness. In developing countries where agricultural work practices and expectations of children differ from

Table 12B.2. Example of modified NAGCAT guidelines for growing and harvesting sugarcane in the Philippines

Tasks	Hazards	Injury/disease concerns	recommended procedures	Training required
Walk to crop field	Slippery, cracked, or uneven surfaces	Scrapes/abrasions, bruises/contusions, and sprains/ strains/ torn ligaments from falls	Rubber shoes/ slippers	Having rubber shoes would be the ideal. However, in the absence of rubber shoes, children should be made aware of the dangers of walking to the field site. These dangers include cracks in the ground and grass-covered irrigation canals.
Bend and cut weeds	Repetitive motion Cutting tools (trowel) Sun Insects	Muscle strain Cuts/lacerations Rubbing from cutting tools Heat exposure Heat exhaustion Insect bites	See NAGCAT's bending guidelines (determine modifications specific to children in the Philippines) Cutting tools are properly sized to the child Leather or moisture-resistant gloves Wear long sleeved shirt, long pants, wide brimmed hat, sunglasses and sunscreen Drink plenty of water Insect repellant	Bending techniques Training on safe use of cutting tools; children should not rush while cutting weeds in order to avoid external injuries. Children should also use shoes and long pants, long sleeves, and gloves to avoid lacerations from cutting tools. Raising awareness on importance of using gloves Raising awareness on heat exposure and exhaustion In tropical climates such as the Philippines, the risk of contracting dengue is increased without the use of repellants
Loosen soil and plant sugarcane	Planting/cutting tools	Cuts/lacerations Punctures/stabs/jabs	Protect feet with shoes/ slippers	Children use the planting or cutting tools to loosen the soil when the cane points are planted. Children also use their feet to plant and secure the cane points in the ground. Children should do this slowly, and wear rubber shoes/slippers when planting the cane points

Carry and apply fertilizer	Weight of container filled with fertilizer Contact with fertilizer	Back strain Rashes and skin diseases	Container should be 10 to 15% of child's body weight (determine modifications specific to children in the Philippines) Moisture-resistant long gloves to cover entire length of arm	Training on harmful effects of handling fertilizer
Bend and cut sugarcane	Cutting (bolo/ cane knife)	*See associated tasks, hazards, and safety recommendations for bending and cutting weeds*		
Carry bunches of sugarcane to trucks	Weight	Back strain Cuts from sugarcane	Weight of sugarcane should be appropriate to individual's body weight and/or should be transported using a carabao drawn cart Protective clothing and gloves Lessen transport distance of sugarcanes from field to truck	Lifting techniques

Source: This job hazard analysis is adapted from various children's tasks outlined by the North American Guidelines for Children's Agricultural Task (NAGCAT) at www.nagcat.org. The author, Dr. Charita Castro, made modifications based on occupational tasks specific to the experiences of the small sample of children working on sugarcane farms in the Philippines [13].

North American practices, further interventions and testing are warranted to assess optimal methods to generate and promote use of guidelines that will have the greatest impact on preventing childhood agricultural injuries.

Acknowledgements

The original North American Guidelines for Children's Agricultural Tasks (NAGCAT) were funded by the National Institute for Occupational Safety and Health, which also funded other NAGCAT- related research and intervention projects. The author extends appreciation to the many people who have studied and applied the guidelines since their development. Gratitude is especially extended to those who have strived to improve working conditions for children in developing countries. Drs. Nathan and Connie Gundaker conducted their work in Mexico. Michele Schermann interacted with Hmong families in Saint Paul, MN and Dr. Charita Libao Castro applied NAGCAT principles in the Philippines.

References

1 Forastieri V (2002). *Children at Work: Health and safety risks*, 2nd ed. Geneva: International Labour Organization.

2 Lessenger JE (2006). *Agricultural Medicine: A practical guide*. New York: Springer Science + Business Media.

3 Commission on Behavioral and Social Sciences and Education (1998). *Protecting Youth at Work: Health, Safety, and Development of Working Children and Adolescents in the United States*. Washington, DC: National Academy Press.

4 Lee B, Marlenga B (1999). *Professional resource manual: North American guidelines for children's agricultural tasks*. Marshfield, WI: Marshfield Clinic.

5 Doty B, Marlenga B (2006). North American guidelines for children's agricultural tasks: Five-year assessment and priorities for the future. *American Journal of Industrial Medicine*, **49**(11):911–9.

6 Hard D (2008). A decade of childhood agricultural health and safety research. Presented at the 6th International Symposium Public Health and the Agricultural Rural Ecosystem. Saskatoon, SK, Canada (abstract 1650).

7 Gadomski A, Ackerman S, Burdick P, Jenkins P (2006). Efficacy of the North American guidelines for children's agricultural tasks in reducing childhood agricultural injuries. *American Journal of Public Health*, **96**(4): 722–7.

8 Miller ME, Fisher R, Lee B, Mulhern B (2008). Safety guidelines for hired adolescent farm workers. Presented at the 136th American Public Health Association Annual Meeting and Exposition. San Diego, CA. Available at http://apha.confex.com/apha/136am/webprogram/Paper187648.html (accessed 31 March 2009).

9 National Children's Center for Rural and Agricultural Health and Safety (2009). Safety guidelines for hired adolescent farm workers. Available at www.marshfieldclinic.org/saghaf (accessed 31 March 2009).

10 U.S. Department of Labor (revised June 2007). Child labor requirements in agricultural occupations under the Fair Labor Standards Act (Child Labor Bulletin 102). Available at http://www.dol.gov/esa/whd/regs/compliance/childlabor102.pdf (accessed 31 March 2009).

11 Rasmussen RC, Schermann MA, Shutske JM, Olson DK (2003). Use of the North American guidelines for children's agricultural tasks with Hmong farm families. *Journal of Agricultural Safety and Health*, **9**(4):265–74.

12 Yang C (2005). In Schermann MA (ed) *Orphan Boy the Farmer* (Tub Ntsuag, Tub ua Teb). Minnesota Agricultural Experiment Station, St. Paul, MN. Available at http://www.extension.umn.edu/distribution/cropsystems/DC8311.html.

13 Castro C (2007). Child sakadas in Philippine agriculture: Researching injury hazards for working children in the context of international labor standards and United States foreign policy. Dissertation. DAI-A 68/04. Available at http://proquest.umi.com/pqdlink?Ver=1&Exp=04-14-2014&FMT=7&DID=1335359961&RQT=309&attempt=1&cfc=1 (accessed 15 April 2009).

Chapter 12C

Illustrative case study C: Traditional communities' rights and child labour: Coco-babaçu workers in Brazil

Noemi Miyasaka Porro and
Anaclaudia G. Fassa

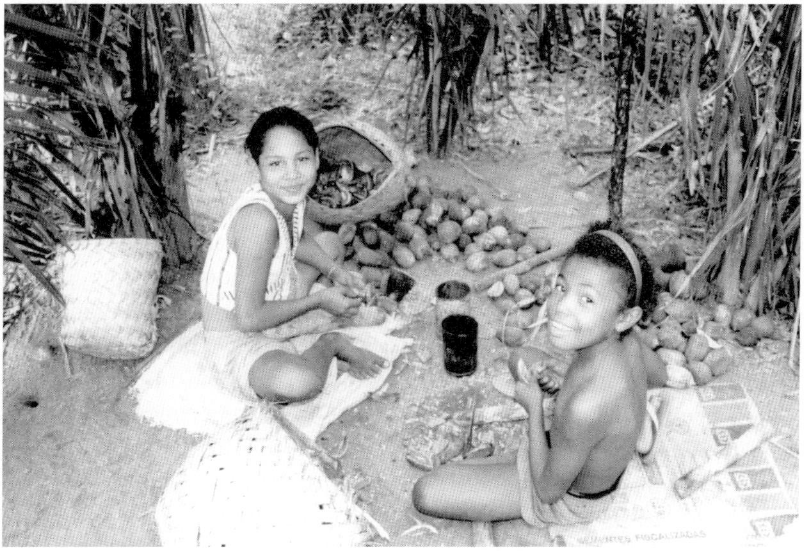

Breaking babaçu palm fruits, Brazil

These authorities issuing such laws...Do they think there are ballet and swimming classes right on the corner for us to send our children, as they can send theirs? ... But the question is not really that... of course no mother wants to have her child with back ache, fingers cut. We want schools and sports right here in the village..., but we need to raise our kids on our own way, because we are the ones who know how is life here. Babaçu breaking is food, brings money, but it is culture too, you know? (Maria Adelina Chagas, babaçu breaker woman, Centro de São José dos Mouras, 2008)

Introduction

This case study is about traditional communities[1] in the Brazilian Amazon, for whom extractive work on babaçu palm forests is the foundation of their social identity and livelihood. It illustrates the tension between an ethnic-based local rights approach to child labour and the wider global human rights approach.

An estimated 400,000 families live on agricultural and extractive activities in 18 million hectares covered by babaçu (*Attalea speciosa*) palm forests in northern and northeastern Brazil [1, 2]. In these communities, babaçu fruits are gathered and kernels are extracted by women and children for domestic consumption, and sale to oil industries for the production of edible oils, soaps, and cosmetics. Agricultural activities are directed by men in small slash-and-burn openings in the forest named *roças*, and the families work in this shifting cultivation, managing agricultural and extractive resources in the palm forests within their traditional territories.

To varying degrees, these traditional communities are an integration of three distinct ethnic groups: detribalized indigenous people, descendants of enslaved Africans, and migrants displaced by landlords from northeastern lands. They have formed a common and unique social identity and way of life. Historically, their social relations with the wider Brazilian society have been antagonistic, and they have developed their own forms of social organization and a distinctive agro-extractive system of economic production in order to survive physically and as a distinct social group with specific ethnic-based rules [3].

In this social organization, what constitutes childhood and what defines child work are strongly informed by their ethnic-based interpretation. Child labour in these communities is intrinsically part of the family unit of production, as a way of ensuring the continuation of their social identity, and as protection against subordination in the context of what they regard as a social struggle. As a result of their work, these communities have managed to conserve extensive babaçu palm forests to support their livelihoods in the Amazon basin [4, 5]. Despite these undeniable social, economic, and environmental achievements, these workers have been excluded from major agrarian and economic policies which favour logging, cattle ranching, and agribusiness for international commodities production. These policies have in turn resulted in wealth and land concentration and in environmental degradation.

[1] Decree 6040/2007 in its Art. 3o. Inc.I defines: 'Traditional peoples and communities are culturally differentiated groups, who recognize themselves as such, and who have their own forms of social organization, occupy and use territories and natural resources as condition for their cultural, social religious, ancestral and economic reproduction, utilizing knowledge, innovations and practices generated and transmitted through tradition'. http://www.planalto.gov.br/CCIVIL/Ato2007-2010/2007/Decreto/D6040.htm

Since the mid-1980s, families who break babaçu fruits to extract kernels have actively participated in collective acts of resistance, especially against the usurpation of their traditional territories and attempts to impose top-down rules that affect their ways of life [6]. The hazards of child labour have been a long-term concern of babaçu breaker women and meetings and workshops on the issue have taken place within their grassroots organizations since 1993. They are culturally aware that children are more vulnerable than adults, and that greater levels of protection are required for the younger family members.

In June of 2008, the Brazilian government ratified ILO Convention 182 through Decree 6.481 [7], about the worst forms of child labour, listing activities such as using blades, excessive weight lifting, charcoal processing, among others. At least 11 of these activities occur as part of the extraction of babaçu resources. In August 2008, the Movement of the Babaçu Breaker Women and the Association in the Settlement Areas in the State of Maranhão hired a safety engineer, an anthropologist, and two epidemiologists to carry out a 'Hazard Mapping Project' concerning child labour in babaçu extractive activities. Hazard mapping is a research process in which the job-related risks are evaluated by the workers through the examination of each step of the work process. In this case, hazard mapping entailed the evaluation of job process from babaçu fruit collection to the processing of its components [8]. This chapter includes information from this Hazard Mapping Project [9] and from ethnographic studies conducted by Porro which describe child labour in the context of babaçu extraction [10].

Child work in the babaçu palm forests

In traditional communities in the babaçu palm forests, within a family unit of production, children are assigned to gender differentiated work activities. Girls are initiated in babaçu breaking, while boys are assigned to what is called *serviço de menino* – 'kids' work', and serve as messengers, carry small loads to *roças* and gather babaçu fruits. As they grow, boys take food to the *roça* and participate in *coivara*– the gathering of unburned slashed branches and trunks and organizing them in rows, and other *roça* activities until they are ready for the heaviest task of slashing at age of 17 or 18 years.

In the 1980s, boys and girls as young as 5 or 6 years old could be observed learning to break open babaçu fruits. Now, as a result of public policies related to food security, poverty alleviation, and eradication of child labour (Cash transfers under the 'Bolsa Família' [11] and the Child Labour Eradication Programme (PETI) [12]), it is estimated that the starting age has risen to around 10 or 11 years. Children are taught to understand economic resources and ecosystems and also develop an understanding of their identity as boys and girls by the way in which labour is assigned. In traditional communities, the work regime is controlled by the family, and in some communities cooperatives and associations have been formed to boost income.

Children accompany their mothers, grandmothers, or older brothers to gather babaçu in the forest. They pick the fruits on the ground and carry them in bags or baskets, or on donkeys back home. To break a babaçu fruit, a worker sits on the ground, the fruit is held over the blade of an axe with the fingers of the left hand. The axe is placed on the ground with its blade up and secured by placing a leg over the handle. The fruit is forced through the blade by the strike of a club held by the right hand and broken in half, and then in quarters or more, freeing the kernels.

From the unripe babaçu fruit, the workers extract the *mesocarp* – a starchy pulp in between the husks and the *endocarp* – the hard inner layer that holds the kernels. This is achieved by soaking the fruit in water for a few minutes, draining it, and then peeling the husks with a machete. Next, the remaining fibers are removed with a knife, the peeled fruit washed and struck with a club to loosen and remove the mesocarp flakes. From the endocarp, once or twice a month, charcoal is made. To make the charcoal, adults and older children dig a hole, build a fire in it and fill it up with babaçu shells. When the shells are on fire, they sprinkle water on top and cover the hole with banana leaves and dirt. Children help to fill the hole with shells and also unload charcoal when it is ready and cold, two days later.

Work-related hazards

The main hazards identified during the Hazard Mapping Project were exposure to sun, heat, and physical hazards, and risk of injuries in the various phases of production. Exposure to dust fumes and noise were also features of activities in communities owning milling machines. In situations when babaçu palms were gathered at a distance from the home, and women and children had to break babaçu in the forest instead of bringing them back home, sun and heat exposure was aggravated by water shortage. This was also a hazard during charcoal production, when heat was increased by fires.

The main physical hazards identified were lifting and carrying heavy loads, while transporting babaçu fruits from gathering sites to the home. Some families carried babaçu fruits on donkeys but others carried the fruits on their shoulders. Children carried what their parents consider adequate. Work in awkward postures and repetitive movements were problems due to frequent bending while babaçu picking, sitting in restricted postures while breaking fruit and the repetitive movements required for this. The basket loaded with kernels was carried on one shoulder, but typically on the top of the head.

Children were exposed to risk of injuries at several stages of the work process: falling babaçu fruit was neither a minor event nor rare; the rough terrain predisposed to falls; children used cutting tools such as machetes and axes. Poisonous animals could also cause accidents during work and travel. Cuts from thorns or babaçu shells also occurred.

During charcoal production, workers were exposed to the risk of burns from hot materials. The filled hole was covered with leaves, and there was a risk that workers would step on a still hot *caieira* if it was not adequately signposted, which was usually done with branches. Babaçu bunches were poked by adults to make fruits to fall from the trees. In this situation children may have been exposed to vegetable dust falling from palm trees. Babaçu husks could also have given off vegetable dust in various phases of the process. Fumes were a potential hazard in charcoal production. These work activities all took place with the family unit, and in those communities which formed the sample for the research, children did not leave school in order to work, but rather combined work activities with their school schedule.

Among babaçu breakers, families work as a unit, and mothers and grandmothers do not have an employer–employee relation with their children. While learning the process of babaçu breaking, children have supervision and care in dealing with risks and preventing accidents. This supervision takes place not only at family level, but also at village level, through a network of neighbours and friends. In some communities, children aged less than 12 years are prohibited from participation during the most hazardous phases of charcoal production, and there are procedures to better control fumes.

An essential feature of these traditional communities is their aversion to 'working for a boss', which is perceived as a form of 'captivity'. The family is responsible for controlling and organizing its own work force. For children, babaçu breaking begins as play and mothers decide how much and how long each child can take part, not only according to age, but also according to individual capabilities. Thus, the working hours and speed of production are flexible and determined by balancing need, capability, and local practices. For example, a teenage girl is not supposed to carry heavy weights or touch metallic cutting tools while menstruating and baskets and other tools are made in different sizes for different children.

Work hazards in the context of daily reality

In traditional economies, local norms and traditions can determine the nature of children's activities within the family unit of production. Such norms might be considered prejudicial [13] and supporters of child labour eradication would argue against children accompanying their parents into the forest to be initiated into babaçu breaking, even in the knowledge that they will not miss school. In this case, local cultural norms are of the view that children are better off in the forests with their parents than at home, where, left alone they might be exposed to other and potentially greater risks. The children who help their parents in the forest, it is argued, learn about family and community work and are better prepared for adult life. Child participation in the family unit of production is viewed as essential for development and socialization, more than just a way to guarantee income, it confers group identity and the maintenance of community values through generations. Children in turn are proud of their activities, which generates positive self-esteem.

Protecting cultural norms may not be sufficient justification for exposing children to hazardous practices. However, in babaçu breaking this work takes place in a context where children's rights to protection and provision are already compromised in several ways. Communities lack basic sanitation and local health services. Elementary schools are part-time, have few resources, and the curriculum is often completely disconnected from local realities. There are neither efficient services for pre-school child care nor middle or high schools within walking distances from villages. Most importantly, many communities still face agrarian conflicts, deforestation, or the consequences of land grabbing, which increases walking distances to palm forests.

These issues all contribute to increase the hazards faced by children. In these communities child activities are not perceived as an issue isolated from the family as a unit of production, which in turn is dependent on the above issues. Thus, work-related hazards cannot be considered in isolation. In fact, child labour eradication may be perceived by these communities as disrespectful of their ethnic identity because it challenges the traditional way in which knowledge is transmitted from one generation to the next and would prejudice the integrity and survival of these communities and their territories. These communities further allege that child labour eradication is in conflict with the right to self-determination by traditional communities as stated in ILO Convention 169 [14], and furthermore that it would infringe on a child's rights to integral protection under the1989 Convention on the Rights of the Child [15].

Conclusions

This case study illustrates the tension that exists between international legislation on child labour, human rights, and ethnic-based local perceptions and practices. ILO Convention 169 assures the right to self-determination by traditional communities, while Conventions 138 [16] and 182 [17] effectively prohibit this sort of child labour. Article 26 of the Universal Declaration of Human Rights [18] affirms that '*Parents have a prior right to choose the kind of education that shall be given to their children*' and, according to ILO, a fundamental principle for the interpretation of the Convention 169 is the consultation and self-determination of the interested peoples. One Convention cannot be subordinated to another. As they were all ratified in Brazil, they entered in the national juridical order at the same hierarchic level. ILO 169 Art 80, Inc 2 affirms:

> These peoples shall have the right to retain their own customs and institutions, where these are not incompatible with fundamental rights defined by the national legal system and with internationally recognised human rights. Procedures shall be established, whenever necessary, to resolve conflicts which may arise in the application of this principle.

Grassroots organizations representing traditional people who have not been adequately consulted on this legislation have demanded the establishment of procedures to resolve these conflicting conceptions, aiming at an effective protection to their children.

As work, education, and childhood all have different meanings according to different ethnic and cultural understanding, the dilemma is how to achieve the goals of both the Universal Declaration of Human Rights and ILO Conventions and, ultimately, protect children's rights to health and education within their own cultures, and within the wider pluri-ethnic societies within which this conflict of values exists.

> Human rights are misconceived if they are understood as a breviary of values: Rights talk can do no more than formalize the terms in which conflicts of values are made precise and therefore rendered amenable to compromise and solution. This is their dynamic: They do not, in themselves, resolve arguments; they create the steadily burgeoning case law, which in turn expands the ambit of human rights claims. [19]

From a rights-oriented public health perspective, ethnic groups' values, such as those of traditional communities, must be better understood. This requires a rupture with 'the monopoly to define rights' that has been established in societies with diverse ethnicities but unbalanced power differentials [20].

In the so-called globalization era, the definition of rights might be assumed to have had a global consensus. However, as this case study illustrates, the perception of these rights varies according to the ethnic-based values of different social groups. Local values may be in conflict with wider societal values that define what children's rights are. At least in Latin America, the national arena is the social space where these conflicts of values can be debated and negotiated [21]. All Nation-States should assure that there is a space where diverse social groups can do the same.

References

1 Almeida AWB (2006). Terras de Quilombo, terras indígenas, 'Babaçuais Livres', 'Castanhais do Povo', Faxinais e Fundos de Pasto: terras tradicionalmente ocupadas Manaus: PPGSCA-UFAM; Ford Foundation.

2 Comunicação Social (1982) Mapeamento e levantamento do potencial das ocorrências de babaçuais nos estados do Maranhão , Piauí, Mato Grosso e Goiás . Brasília: MIC.

3 Almeida AWB, Mourão L (1979). Questões agrárias no Maranhão contemporâneo. Belém: Universidade Federal do Pará, Editora Universitária.

4 Anderson AB, May P, Balick MJ (1991). The subsidy from nature: palm forests, peasantry, and development on an Amazon frontier. New York: Columbia University Press.

5 May P (1990). Palmeiras em chamas: transformação agrária e justiça social na Zona do Babaçu. São Luís: EMAPA, FINEP, Fundação Ford.

6 Porro NM (2002). Rupture and resistance: gender relations and life trajectories in the Babaçu Palm Forests of Brazil [Ph.D. Dissertation]. Gainesville: University of Florida.

7 Brasil, Congresso Nacional (2008). Decree-Law no. 6.481/2008. Hazardous Child Labor. Brasília: República Federativa do Brasil.

8 Laurell AC, Noriega M, López O, Martínez S, Ríos V, Vllegas J (1989). Manual conocer para cambiar: estudio de la salud en el trabajo. Mexico: Universidad Autónoma Metropolitana Xochimilco.

9 Mapping of Hazards Project. Research funded by ILO Brazil. [Unpublished manuscript proposed by the Movement of the Babaçu Breaker Women]. Contact assessoria@miqcb.org.br.

10 Porro NM (1997). Changes in peasant perceptions of conservation and development [Master Thesis]. Gainesville: Florida University.

11 Brasil, Ministério do Desenvolvimento Social e Combate à Fome (MDS) (2004). Law no. 10.836, of 9 January 2004. Creates the 'Programa Bolsa Família' and other provisions. Brasilia: República Federativa do Brasil.

12 Brasil (2000). Ordinance no. 2.917, of 12 September 2000. Establishes guidelines for PETI. Brasilia: República Federativa do Brasil.

13 Shiraishi Neto J (2006). Leis do Babaçu Livre: práticas jurídicas das quebradeiras de Coco Babaçu e normas correlatas. Manaus: UFAM, Fundação Ford.

14 International Labor Organization (ILO) (1989). Convention 169. Convention concerning Indigenous and Tribal Peoples in Independent Countries. Geneva: ILO.

15 United Nations (1989). Convention on the Rights of the Child.

16 International Labor Organization (ILO) (1973). Convention 138. Convention concerning minimum age for admission to employment. Geneva: ILO.

17 International Labor Organization (ILO) (1999). Convention 182. Convention concerning the Prohibition and Immediate Action for the Elimination of the Worst Forms of Child Labour. Geneva: ILO.

18 United Nations (1948). Universal Declaration of Human Rights. Article 26.

19 Ignatieff M (1999). Human rights. In Hesse C, Post R (eds), *Human Rights in Political Transition:From Gettysburg to Bosnia*, pp. 313–24. New York: Zone Books.

20 Bourdieu P(1989). A força do direito: Elementos para uma sociologia do campo jurídico. In Bourdieu P,(ed.) *O poder simbólico*, pp. 209–54. Lisboa: Difel.

21 Escobar A (2001). Place, economy, and culture in a post-development era. In Prazniak R, Dirlik A (eds), *Places and Politics in an Age of Globalization*, pp. 193–218. Boulder, CO: Rowman & Littlefield Publishers.

Part 4

Conclusions

Chapter 13

Child labour and health: Changing the future

Anaclaudia G. Fassa, David L. Parker, and Thomas J. Scanlon

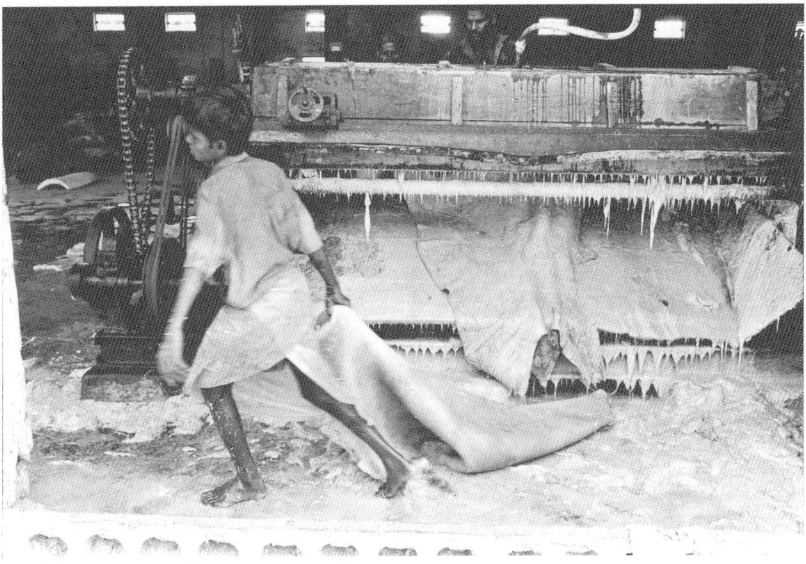

Leather tanning, India

Introduction

Public health has been defined as 'the science and art of preventing disease, prolonging life and promoting health through the organized efforts and informed choices of society, organizations, public and private, communities and individuals'. [1] This final chapter summarizes the key findings that have emerged from an examination of a rights-oriented public health model of child labour, considers what comprises appropriate child work and makes recommendations for further action to more effectively address child labour.

Key findings from the rights-oriented public health approach

Epidemiology

There are numerous datasets on child labour, each established for a slightly different purpose and compiled in a different manner. This causes some confusion as to the nature and extent of child labour around the world [2–4]. Many countries do not have accurate information on child labour. Nevertheless, it is clear that child labour represents a scourge on the lives of over 200 million children aged 5 to 14 years across the globe, particularly those living in sub-Saharan Africa and Asia.

Child labour data are becoming more comprehensive and more accurate. With this comes the ability to monitor trends and the impact of intervention programmes. Better data also make it possible to harness the political and public support required to comprehensively tackle child labour.

Economics

At a macro-economic level there is a strong association between a nation's economic status and the economic activity of children. Child labour is widespread in poor economies but unusual in more wealthy countries. The variation between countries in the gross domestic product per capita has been found to explain almost three quarters of the variation in the economic activities of children [5]. However, countries with different gross domestic products differ in many other ways associated with child labour including, the availability of education, health and social care, legislative infrastructure, and social values.

At a micro-economic level there is a strong association between household poverty and child labour. In Nepal, children have been estimated to be responsible for 9% of the gross national product [6]. As is the case at the macro-economic level, one of the problems in determining to what degree this is a causal relationship is the fact that poor households differ from rich households in many different ways that are associated with child labour. One approach to gaining a broader understanding has been to track families over time, and such studies have almost universally demonstrated that child labour increases when family income declines.

Independent of human rights and public health, a market-led case can be made for government action on hazardous child labour. Working children and their parents often fail to recognize the risks children face when they enter the labour market. Subsequent injury and illness mean the children's lifetime productivity is much reduced. If work exacerbates the spread of illnesses such as tuberculosis or HIV into the community, then further costs will be borne by society.

Initiatives which alleviate poverty and invest in human capital such as conditional cash transfer programmes show considerable promise in terms of reducing poverty and income inequality, improving health and educational outcomes, and reducing child labour. Such programmes have been implemented in Brazil, Guatemala, and Bangladesh with some success. In Mexico, the PROGRESA (later Oportunidades) programme has assisted over 24 million people in the lowest 20% of income distribution. The programme has been particularly noteworthy in that it has successfully targeted girls and in particular girls' access to school through a differential stipend for boys and girls linked to school attendance [7].

Education

The importance of education in addressing child labour cannot be overstated. At the individual level, the availability of child-friendly and high-quality education promotes school attendance and reduces participation in work. Educated children are more likely to be successful as adults in the labour market. Adult educational and employment success has important economic, public health (e.g. reduced maternal mortality) and quality of life benefits for families and communities. Investment in education has the potential to foster a virtuous cycle whereby better educated parents are more likely to forego their children's labour and encourage full-time school attendance [8].

The responsibility of the international community and national governments to improve school facilities and standards, and to lower the costs of schooling are important component parts of achieving this virtuous cycle. Measures to improve the educational infrastructure need to go hand-in-hand with raising awareness among parents and communities of the long-term benefits of investing in their children's education.

Social values

The role of social and cultural values in sustaining children's work is beginning to be recognized within the child labour literature, in policy and in practice. It is evident that cultures vary in their conceptions about how children develop and learn, and place differing emphasis on the contributions children make to their families and communities. Children's involvement in work, whether hazardous or not, may be understood as an important mechanism through which children are integrated into their communities and their transition to adulthood, as well as for the acquisition of skills considered necessary to ensure basic survival [9].

In some communities, work is an integral part of community identity. In such circumstances, any challenge to the continuation of child labour may be regarded as a challenge to that identity. The enforcement of child labour legislation may then be perceived by those communities as capitulation and subordination in the context of what is regarded as a social struggle [10].

An understanding of the social and cultural contexts in which children's work takes place is therefore essential in developing interventions. This does not mean a simple acceptance of hazardous labour because it is socially or culturally sanctioned. Rather, it means that an acknowledgement of the place of child labour in community identity, and a realization that attempts at legislative enforcement, in the face of economic hardship, poor educational opportunities, inadequate health and social care infrastructure, and community opposition are likely to be counter-productive.

Health

As with many other facets of child labour there is an absence of good quality research on the impact of work on the health of children. A number of measures could improve the available evidence base. The first step is improving the quality of research with specific groups of child workers. This requires better sampling, more appropriate control groups, and more accurate identification and monitoring of hazards and outcomes over longer periods of time. These methodological failings have been recognized for some time. They are in large part a consequence of the practical difficulties in studying the health effects of child labour.

Using data from studies undertaken in more developed countries where routine data collection is much more complete can shed light on the health effects of child labour in less economically developed countries. This is perhaps best exemplified by the data on work-related injuries in children and young people, most of which comes from the United States and Canada [11].

Data on the psychosocial function and social/intellectual developmental (PSID) effects of child labour are most notable by their absence. One of the reasons for this absence has been that PSID effects comprise a constellation of conditions such as mental illness, addiction, and stress. Research tools have not been available to assess these problems in working children. Researchers are now working to define a framework that identifies the major psychosocial hazards. For the time being, however, these effects remain largely under-recorded.

Studies of children who do not work but who are exposed through the environment to particular hazards can provide insight into the health of working children. Similarly, studies of adults who are exposed to hazards through their occupations can contribute to the knowledge base. There are caveats with such data; environmental exposure is different from work exposure, adults differ from children in many physiological respects and children differ from one another substantially at different stages of development. Regardless, to ignore existing data while undertaking robust child labour specific studies in developing countries remains so challenging, is to miss an opportunity.

It is a contention of this book that the health impact of child labour should be considered with regard to both its immediate and long-term effects on the child, as well as its impact on the community. The wider effects on the community from child labour and vice versa, such as infections like tuberculosis and HIV are rarely examined. Disentangling which exposures in communities are as a consequence of child labour and which stem from other environmental sources is likely to be problematic. Until the child labour literature considers these wider family and community effects, only part of the child labour and health story will be told.

Legislation

There is a wide range of international legislation addressing child labour. In recent years, child labour policy has moved from prohibition and minimum age requirements to the elimination of the worst forms of child labour and the identification and elimination of hazardous child labour. This has been demonstrated by the reduced focus on ILO (Minimum Age) Convention 138 and the increased focus on ILO (Elimination of the Worst Forms of Child Labour) Convention 182. However, Convention 182 still maintains some focus on age through the requirement of signatories to construct hazardous child labour lists: age is generally considered a key feature in the identification of hazardous child work.

Assessing the impact of legislation is difficult and ratification says little or nothing about national and local enforcement. In fact, some states openly ratify treaties with statements limiting their applicability within those countries. In the face of long-established local practices, where previous child labour laws may have come and gone, legislation alone is likely to have little impact.

Child labour legislation may be most effective in terms of its role as a stimulus for social change. In this respect, it serves as a tool to raise awareness and assists in placing child labour high on the agenda of national and local governments, rather than in terms of sanctions or punitive impact. The country-wide case studies in this book provide good evidence that where individual countries have adopted comprehensive measures to address child labour, the enactment and enforcement of national legislation has been important in raising awareness, gaining momentum, and in harnessing a high-level commitment to change [12].

Another important role of legislation, as exemplified by Convention 182, is the creation and adoption of hazardous child labour lists [13, 14]. This is examined in more detail in the context of appropriate child work later in this chapter.

Rights

The over-arching domain of human rights is a key principle of this model of child labour. All children have the rights to be protected and to be provided for, although for many children across the world these rights are breached on a daily basis.

The right of children and communities to participate in addressing child labour is often inadvertently overlooked. Measures to address child labour, which may comprise commendable initiatives to build human capital, reduce poverty, provide educational opportunities, and improve public health infrastructure are likely to fall short if the participation of children and communities is overlooked.

Children and communities have the right to participate in the identification and implementation of solutions to the problems they face. This is a fundamental requirement with practical consequences and provides a sound basis for research and public health practice. If children and communities actively participate in finding and implementing solutions, these solutions are much more likely to be sustainable.

Appropriate child work

Convention 182 states that the types of work to be considered hazardous shall be determined by national laws. The development of a list of hazardous child labour should take place in consultation with employers, workers, and public health officials [13]. According to the accompanying Recommendation 190 [14] consideration should be given to:

1. Work which exposes children to physical, psychological, or sexual abuse;
2. Work underground, under water, at dangerous heights or in confined spaces;
3. Work with dangerous machinery, equipment and tools, or which involves the manual handling or transport of heavy loads;
4. Work in an unhealthy environment which may, for example, expose children to hazardous substances, agents or processes, or to temperatures, noise levels, or vibrations damaging to their health;
5. Work under particularly difficult conditions such as work for long hours or during the night or work where the child is unreasonably confined to the premises of the employer.

Hazardous child labour lists are required to be periodically reviewed and revised; this is an acknowledgement that these lists will have a context which is both cultural and contemporaneous.

As previously discussed, classifying child labour as hazardous is a complex task. Some work has the potential to be a positive experience and the published literature on child labour and health is limited. Despite these difficulties, there are sufficient data if adult studies or studies of exposures in non-working children are used to support the development of hazardous child labour lists.

There are a number of approaches to the development of hazardous child labour lists, which are not all encompassing, nor mutually exclusive. Approaches may focus on occupations, tasks, and conditions of work within specific occupations, related hazards and their associated tasks.

The examination of risks may offer the best theoretical option for establishing a hazardous child labour list. This is particularly true if three key criteria can be assessed,

1 The magnitude of the problem: the number of children exposed to the activity;

2 The probability of harm to health;

3 The severity of the potential harm.

Any of these three criteria may lead to a conclusion that a problem needs to be addressed. For example, a less serious problem may affect large numbers of children. Conversely, a more serious problem may affect few children but have dire consequences.

The second and third criteria, the probability of harm and the severity of harm, need to be considered in the context of the specific vulnerability of children, i.e., the features of children that mean that their vulnerability is different from adults. The identification of age-appropriate work implies a defining of unacceptable risk. In general, work becomes increasingly harmful the younger the age of the child and the greater the impact on education, recreation, and rest, as well as long-term growth and development. Cut-off points are difficult to identify and are contemporaneous. The prevailing view on what constitutes appropriate work today is more restrictive than it was in the previous decades.

No work exists without some element of risk and hazardous child labour lists should not seek to catalogue every conceivable task or activity. A hazardous child labour list should have the primary purpose of defining a level of unacceptable risk. A limited list has the advantage of enabling programmes of eradication to be better targeted.

Many countries have looked to ILO for support in order to construct hazardous child labour lists in line with the Convention 182. To provide a stimulus for the development of hazardous child labour lists, the ILO set up a meeting of experts [15]. One of the proposals of this group was a 'zero-exposure list', which defined activities or exposures considered totally unacceptable for children in all countries. The zero-exposure list included several chemical exposures and a number of activities such as working underground or at high temperatures.

Another proposal was the development of lists in a matrix format. This is accomplished by listing occupations, job tasks, associated hazards, and their potential outcomes. The matrix format also serves as a tool to educate workers and community members about potential risks from different types of employment.

The systematic identification of hazardous work activities based on empirical evidence should be encouraged. This may be accomplished through a combination of methods depending on the resources available. Methods include household surveys, rapid assessments of communities or industries, analysis of hazards, and surveillance programmes. However, some caution is required to ensure that risks are clearly understood in the context of both short- and long-term effects as well as their impact on communities. External technical support may be required where local expertise is not available. For countries with limited resources, this flexible approach could also assist in focusing attention on the most hazardous industries that deserve immediate attention.

Conclusions and recommendations

Children who have been trafficked or are in armed conflict; forced or bonded labour; prostitution or pornography; or other illicit work activities such as drug trafficking, should be freed from these unconditional worst forms of child labour as soon as possible. However, there remains the challenge of identifying which other groups of children are being harmed by their work.

Simple eradication of all children's work is not currently an option. The impact of child labour on health varies and considerable research remains to be done on linking work of different intensities, at particular ages and with regard to gender and socioeconomic circumstances to different outcomes. The harm that children experience manifests itself in many guises with acute, latent, and chronic effects on the child and the wider community. Work that is identified as harmful should be addressed so that either the hazards are eliminated or sufficiently mitigated, or the work is halted. Measures taken to address harm should be undertaken with the community rather than on the community.

Better information is required to tackle child labour and some improvements could be made at little cost. Incidence and prevalence data are poor and exposure and health outcome data are lacking. National household surveys could be amended to capture information on the prevalence of work, the incidence of injury and other health outcomes. With additional research, data collection could be extended to include information on the psychological, social, and developmental effects of child labour. The ability to identify and measure hazardous work more accurately would assist in advancing better targeted interventions, and would help with wider societal efforts to prevent child labour in the first place.

Interventions which build human capital and reduce poverty, such as conditional cash transfers, probably offer the greatest impact on child labour. These, however, need to be linked to more comprehensive programmes which tackle social values, public health infrastructure, legislation, and education.

The development, adoption, and enforcement of hazardous child labour lists, offers a practical way forward. These lists can make explicit to employers and employees alike what is appropriate and acceptable, and what is not. They also help to focus the efforts of different agencies, statutory and non-governmental, seeking to eradicate hazardous child labour. To date, hazardous child labour lists have been subject to little if any formal evaluation in terms of their impact. As hazardous child labour lists represent a potential legislative arm in the effort to eliminate hazardous child labour, implementation efforts should be tied to evaluation.

The ILO/IPEC time bound programmes have been an important part of international efforts to address child labour in recent years. It is clear that these initiatives are meant to be a stimulus for comprehensive national action and not a substitute. The case study from Kenya, however, illustrates how it was ILO/IPEC that provided the leadership for addressing child labour and not the national government. An important role of ILO/IPEC is not to replace or compensate for government failings, but rather to engage at the right level of seniority within government.

A lack of national and local leadership has implications for the adoption and sustainability of comprehensive measures to address child labour. In both Kenya and the Philippines, a range of policies and programmes of action were established. Regardless, without strong leadership in Kenya there was weak enactment and enforcement. In the Philippines where initiatives were dependent upon project funding, there was no sustainability.

The effort and commitment required to address child labour in very poor nations should not be underestimated. Where leadership, commitment, and funding can be secured and where a comprehensive approach that addresses education, poverty, social values, and legislation is adopted, considerable progress can be made. This is demonstrated by the more successful approaches taken in Brazil and Mexico.

This book has offered the reader a rights-oriented public health perspective on child labour. It is clear that compared to the work of adults, the work of children is overlooked and important opportunities are lost for children, their families, and communities.

Significant progress has been made over the past decade. With a greater understanding of the causes and consequences of child labour, there is hope for greater success in implementing the sustainable solutions that working children and their communities deserve.

References

1 Winslow CEA (1920) The untilled fields of public health, *Science*, **50**.

2 International Labour Office (2008). Report III, Child labour statistics. Geneva: International Labour Organization.

3 UNICEF. Statistics and Monitoring: Multiple Indicator Cluster Surveys (MICS). (n.d.) Geneva.

4 The World Bank. Living Standards Measurement Study. The World Bank; (n.d.)

5 Edmonds E (2008). Child labor, In Schultz TP, Strauss J (eds), *Handbook of Development Economics*, Vol. 4, pp. 3607–710. Amsterdam: Elsevier Science.

6 Menon M, Pareli F, Rosati F (2005). Estimation of the contribution of child labour to the formation of rural incomes: An application to Nepal. Working Paper no. 10. Rome, Italy: Centre for Household Income, Labour, and Demographic Economics.

7 Emmanuel Skoufias E, Parker S, Behrman J, Pessino C (2001). Conditional cash transfers and their impact on child work and schooling: Evidence from the PROGRESA program in Mexico. *Economía*, 2:45–96.

8 Mirowsky J, Ross CE (1998). Education, personal control, lifestyle and health: A human capital hypothesis. *Research on Aging*, **20**(4):415–49.

9 Woodhead M (2001). The value of work and school: A study of children's perspectives. In Lieten C, White B (eds), *Child Labour. Policy Options*. Amsterdam: Aksant.

10 Liebel M (2004). *A Will of their Own. Cross-cultural Perspectives on Working Children*. London: Zed Books.

11 National Institute for Occupational Safety and Health (2003). NIOSH Alert: Preventing deaths injuries and illnesses of young workers. Washington, DC: US Department of Health and Human Services.

12 ILO/IPEC (2003): Taking stock of achievements and lessons learned. A Report of a Review of IPEC action against child labour in Kenya 1992–2002, ILO/IPEC Office, Nairobi, Kenya.

13 Convention Concerning the Prohibition and Immediate Action for the Elimination of the Worst Forms of Child Labor (ILO no. 182), 2133 U.N.T.S.161, entered into force 19 November 2000.

14 International Labour Organization Recommendation (no. 190) Concerning Worst Forms of Child Labour Convention, 1999, 17 June 1999, Geneva, Switzerland.

15 Eijkemans G (2002). Final Report of the Preparatory Expert Meeting on Hazardous Child Labour: A Joint ILO (IPEC and Safework) and WHO Consultation. Geneva: International Labour Organization.

Index